Assessment of Practice Performance in
Medicine: A Clinician's Guide to Quality Improvement

Assessment of Practice Performance in Emergency Medicine: A Clinician's Guide to Quality Improvement

Anthony Ferroggiaro, *MD, MHA, FACEP*

New York   Chicago   San Francisco   Athens   London   Madrid
Mexico City   Milan   New Delhi   Singapore   Sydney   Toronto

Assessment of Practice Performance in Emergency Medicine: A Clinician's Guide to Quality Improvement, First Edition

1 2 3 4 5 6 7 8 9 0 CTP/CTP 20 19 18 17 16 15

ISBN 978-0-071-83659-3
MHID 0-07-183659-4

This book was set in Minion Pro by MPS Limited.
The Editors were Brian Belval and Brian Kearns.
The production supervisor was Richard Ruzycka.
Production management was provided by Asheesh Ratra of MPS Limited.
China Translation & Printing Services, Ltd. was printer and binder.

This book is printed on acid-free paper.

Library of Congress Cataloging-in-Publication Data

Ferroggiaro, Anthony, author.
     Assessment of practice performance in emergency medicine : a clinician's
guide to quality improvement / Anthony Ferroggiaro, .
          p. ; cm.
Includes bibliographical references.
Summary: "Improve patient outcomes and meet MOC Part IV requirements with this
real-world guide to implementing quality assessment and practice performance in
emergency medicine. Assessment of Practice Performance in Emergency Medicine delivers
a comprehensive, engagingly written review of our current methods for outcome assessment
and clinical efficacy. The author, an experienced Emergency Department physician, also offers
an insightful, thought-provoking call for a more aggressive, comprehensive, and local process.
Highlights of coverage include: The Standard Peer Chart Review Process, Sequential Clinical
Auditing, Assessment of Practice Performance, Implementing a Sequential Clinical Auditing
Program, Case Studies in Peer Review, Examples of Clinical Audits, Examples and Templates
for compliance with the APP PCPI Component, Integration of these elements in a holistic
physician performance program, How this process can be initiated within your organization,
Essential for every medical director, chairperson, administrator, or physician who is searching
for methods to raise and/or sustain their own technical quality or that of their group,
Assessment of Practice Performance in Emergency Medicine provides a critically
important tool in today's medicine and healthcare market."—Provided by publisher.
ISBN 978-0-07-183659-3 (paperback : alk. paper)—ISBN 0-07-183659-4 (paperback : alk. paper)
I. Title.
[DNLM: 1.   Emergency Medicine—methods. 2.   Outcome Assessment
(Health Care)—methods. 3.   Quality Assurance, Health Care—methods.
WB 105]
RC86.7
616.02′5—dc23
                                                                                                    2015011943

To Michelle, Anna, Sarah, and Thomas

Table of Contents

Chapter 4

Chapter 5

Chapter 6

Preface

Like many young physicians in health care leadership, I started out wanting to change the activity of medicine and was quickly, ironically ... promoted.

My first forays into physician performance were completing peer chart reviews and writing guidelines, then joining hospital peer review groups, then leading quality councils and health system committees. Along the way, I obtained many merit badges, CMEs, and some vision.

I see imbalance; a system shifting on a scale.

In this era of quality and patient safety in health care, I have marveled at the added complexity of the quality and patient safety effort brought to the system but was not surprised when the outcomes were not statistically affirming. I have watched the well-meaning core measures overshoot the evidence and the reactive response of a health system to a Joint Commission visit or waning Hospital Compare score.

I have been subjected to the drive of health care business and customer satisfaction goals. I found myself explaining to nonmedical personnel why I refused to prescribe 40 tablets of Percocet to a drug-seeking patient. I had naïvely considered our goal was limiting community drug addiction and not an unacknowledged method of customer retention.

Working within employed health systems, contract management groups, private practices, as well as academic institutions, I learned much about the physician perspective and behavior. Within those groups, I suffered some challenges developing this model but I was also encouraged with the hopefulness and patient alignment that our profession has retained.

This book offers one answer to correct the imbalance between the current quality and patient safety system, the business of health care and patient satisfaction metrics, and technical medical care. It tries to reduce activity to the local level and empower physicians to manage their craft, outcomes, group, and career.

Anthony Ferroggiaro, MD
May 4, 2015

Assessment of Practice Performance in Emergency Medicine: A Clinician's Guide to Quality Improvement

CHAPTER 1

The Assumption of Clinical Quality

Brothers and sisters,

One evening, I entered an emergency department to start a night shift. The day physician, signing out to me, was quite pleased with himself. He said,

I saw about 30 patients in triage in 2 hours... I bet I missed something.

The emergency department leadership had developed a policy of treating and discharging patients from the waiting room. Understanding that this department is much like others in which patient satisfaction has been aggressively promoted and operationally processes had been developed to achieve this interpretation of patient value, it did not shock me that this physician had given up on accuracy or correctness and had just focused on speed. Ironically, he was achieving a skewed interpretation of the Institute of Medicine aims.[1] I wondered how many patients would be harmed through his "efficiency," his "timeliness," his "concern" for the patient, for "his patient centeredness," and how the patients' "perception" of care would change when they found out their renal function was compromised from a quickly prescribed drug, a missed diagnosis or that they started bleeding from a toxic INR level. I doubted that the administration was monitoring the "return to the ED" rate.

I no longer work there...

As I started writing this appeal I realized that the term, assumption, with its dual meaning had strong linkage to our concerns.

Out of the dictionary,[2] "assumption" is the "thinking that something is true such as a fact or statement" and "taken for granted." A good example in today's health care world is the assumption that physicians provide highly accurate and precise care. People, patients, and families hope, believe, and delude themselves with this idea; physicians often do as well. Rarely do emergency physicians know whether they are 80% successful managing this process or another; the fact is that they might or might not but usually we do not have data to support any conclusion—good or bad.

Another assumption is that physicians are constantly improving their care, technique decay is minimal, and they do not need or they already have adequate programs or processes to assist with improvement. The current processes for maintenance of practice quality are mostly self-directed and have minimal thresholds for compliance.

A third assumption is that patients cannot determine technical quality and that patient satisfaction is a reasonable surrogate marker for technical accuracy and ability.

Still, assumption can be positive.

As this book provides, we can "take [the responsibility of clinical accuracy, outcomes and improvement] to or upon oneself" especially since we are primarily if not solely responsible for these results and can be the only authority for review and action. Similarly, assumption is "the act of laying claim to or taking possession of something" and in this case, as I advocate in the text, we as physicians must continue to "lay claim" to clinical outcomes due to our technical nature and role in health care.

This book is about "hard" quality; the aggressive, at times, uncomfortable look at our practice, our knowledge, our outcomes, and our true technical quality. The currently used hard components of clinical quality do not achieve the goal of assessing overall technical physician performance; there is an incomplete, imbalanced description, review, and management of physician practice (Figure 1-1). Today this void has been filled with assessments of personality and soft quality not to be equated with professionalism or technical competence.

A simple overall view of emergency department activity includes operational management, clinical technical accuracy and effectiveness, and patient satisfaction (Figure 1-2). None of the three foci function in isolation and often overlap with activity. Operational management is about connecting the patient to and from the physician and enacting the physician's decision making. Patient satisfaction activity is about assessing the service delivery with the visit and whether the patient will promote the physician and facility to future patients. Clinical technical accuracy and effectiveness is the activity of those providing care; knowledge base, decision making, and technical ability; represented as practice performance. As stated, there can be overlap; the operational goal of timeliness to cardiac catherizations is linked to effective treatment in STEMI patients. Clinical accuracy and effectiveness, such as a properly anesthetized digit, that results in a pain-free repair is more satisfying to the patient with a finger laceration.

Many physicians are struggling with this health care model. They are trying to comply with the business side of this exchange but realize that the balance is hard

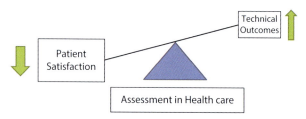

FIGURE 1-1. The imbalance in health care between patient satisfaction and technical outcomes.

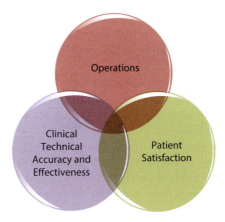

FIGURE 1-2. Simple view of emergency department activity.

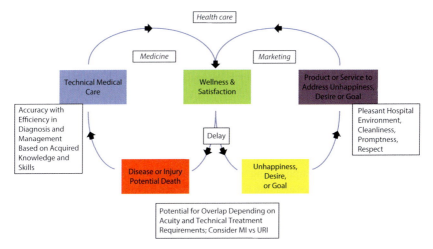

FIGURE 1-3. Simplified relationship between medical care and marketing—technical accuracy emphasis.

to achieve. Medical marketing and outcome medicine can be complementary and not antagonistic. Bowers and Kiefe[3] promote a model showing it is "conceptually feasible to integrate medical and marketing approaches to quality...." Within this model is technical quality associated with outcomes, "hard" quality, as a component *independent* to patient satisfaction and service delivery (Figure 1-3). Further the authors describe service delivery as based on the interaction between the physician and the patient (I would add the organization and the patient) and which contains elements—reliability, responsiveness, assurance, empathy, and the tangibles (physical environment). Bowers and Kiefe state that consumers attempt to assess technical quality but that technical quality may not be directly, overtly obvious to the patient who then must use indirect measures of physician technical competency; "… consumers attempt to use both components when making quality judgments, but if lacking ability to assess technical quality the entire quality judgment is made on delivery quality elements."

If technical quality is not promoted aggressively but instead is a gap or vacuum in the overall concept of health care quality, then other factors of service dominate and the goals can become distorted. If no one but medical professionals can assess technical quality, then (1) we should not allow others to define it or proceed to assess, including patients, and (2) we should be vigorously pursuing systems and programs that promote technical quality and appropriately represent physician technical activity in the model of service delivery and health care process.

This is an appeal to focus on or to assume the technical quality in emergency medicine and in medicine in general; to return to a focus on clinical outcomes, to emphasize that as a team player in a health system, as a physician, your main job is to be clinically the best technician with increasingly higher technical knowledge and skill. This is recognition of the priority function that no one else can do and is required to balance the health care quality process.

In the next five chapters, this book reviews our current methods for outcome assessment and clinical accuracy and advances a more aggressive, comprehensive, local process. In Chapter 2, the standard peer chart review (PCR) process for emergency medicine will be described. We will examine the TJC FPPE and OPPE requirements and structure as a starting point, leading to a more specific discussion on common emergency medicine peer review. I will present a comparison between isolated peer review and a group review process including the incorporation of EBM as a foundation for work comparison. There will be a description of a best method to approach the involved physician as well as a delineation of the "art" of peer review emphasizing a balance of advocacy for the physician and the patient. Several cases and one response letter are included as examples.

Chapter 3 will discuss clinical auditing and specifically sequential clinical auditing (SCA). The latter is work that I have provided to emergency medicine groups, both community and academic, for several years. In comparison to peer review, clinical auditing is disease-specific or chief complaint–specific comprehensive practice review, linked or grounded in evidence-based medicine, in which all the physicians within the group are reviewed simultaneously. Combined as a sequence of audits in a comprehensive program, audits provide a more holistic, accurate view of a physician's and a group's clinical performance. Sequential clinical auditing is one system answer that can be embedded within a larger effort of hospital, practice, and/or department quality improvement as a necessary complement to flow process improvement, patient safety measures, including a way to balance the focus on patient satisfaction. The discussion will show how core measure work, standard peer review, and the new ABEM requirements of practice assessment can be incorporated into this system. This chapter will provide the steps of the process, from selection of topics to the politics of intervention and provide many examples (potentially worth copying) of completed audits.

Chapter 4 will be a discussion on the fourth component of ABEM's maintenance of certification: the assessment of practice performance. This is a new requirement for board-certified emergency physicians and is composed of two sections: "The ABEM APP Patient Care Practice Improvement Requirement" and "The ABEM APP Communication/Professionalism Requirement." I will attempt to describe the components of the requirements with reliance on the ABEM sources in order to assist the curious or concerned emergency physician reader. The PCPI discussion will emphasize an individual clinical focus on the choice of review topics rather than the ABEM-advocated operational topics. Templates for individual completion are provided. In the Communication/Professionalism (C/P) Requirement section, I promote a separation of professionalism from patient satisfaction through a focus on technical quality. The focus will be on components of the physician-patient interaction that enable accuracy of diagnosis, relief of symptoms, and adherence to a treatment plan. The discussion's second half will break down the C/P requirement into categories with direction on methods of completion for the benefit of the individual physician practice.

Chapter 5 will describe how all of these elements can be linked within a physician performance process and how this process can be started within your organization. The emphasis of implementing a program in your group is based on the individual to group dynamic: The group must support the individual such that the individual can support the group. I will discuss different statuses of groups and their readiness for cultural change. Developing a coalition of key influential and power level physicians is invaluable to moving the audit program forward and we will explore which physicians in the group should compose the coalition. I present the mechanics of breaking inertia and monitoring the group process and rate of acceptance as well as the potential organizational impediments to program development and continuance.

This work is written for any medical director, chairperson, administrator, or physician who is searching for methods to raise and/or sustain his or her own technical quality or his/her group's technical quality. This text can be a platform for initiating your work or your program. Though all examples are for emergency medicine, the methods are universal. It is my hope that once you have completed your first read, you feel I argued well for our profession and for a better way.

Anthony Ferroggiaro, MD

REFERENCES

1. Institute of Medicine. *Crossing the quality chasm*. Washington, DC: National Academy Press; 2001.

2. Merriam-Webster. *Webster's ninth new collegiate dictionary*. Springfield, MA: Merriam-Webster; 1983.

3. Bowers MR, Kiefe CI. Measuring health care quality: comparing and contrasting the medical and the marketing approaches. *Am J Med Qual*. 2002;17(4):136-144.

Peer Chart Review

A 2009 survey of hospital leaders[1] on the process of peer review in US hospitals found that the majority of sites (96%) completed retrospective chart review. This was the most frequent and consistent method of peer review identified and probably is a response to regulatory demand and compliance. This chapter will describe the current requirements for and general technique of retrospective chart or case peer review as a comparative background for the clinical auditing chapter (Chapter 3).

■ HOSPITAL PEER REVIEW

Whether individual physicians are specifically aware, each medical staff at every hospital with The Joint Commission (TJC) certification and/or accreditation is required to have a structured peer review process for new applicant physicians requesting privileges and for established physicians requesting a change in or additional privileges. The hospital must have a similar process for ongoing practice evaluation in order to determine appropriateness of continuance of privileges.

■ **TABLE 2-1.** The Joint Commission OPPE and FPPE Focus

Program	Focus
Focused Professional Practice Evaluation (FPPE)	Primary use: New MD privilege specific competence New or change in practice requests with established MD—new techniques, equipment, or provision of service Secondary use: Questions of quality and safety of care identified with OPPE
Ongoing Professional Practice Evaluation (OPPE)	Continue, limit, or revoke privileges

Data from Ref. 2.

TJC titled these processes FPPE and OPPE: Focused Professional Practice Evaluation (FPPE) and Ongoing Professional Practice Evaluation (OPPE).[2] (Table 2-1). Most frequently, the FPPE process is used when "the organization evaluates the privilege-specific competence of the practitioner who does not have documented evidence of competently performing the requested privilege at the organization."[2] This is the expected process in which a medical staff evaluates a new colleague starting to practice at the hospital. The process is also inclusive of any new privilege requested of established physicians, in the case of new techniques, equipment, or provision of service. The secondary use of FPPE is "when a question arises regarding a currently privileged practitioner's ability to provide safe, high quality patient care." The secondary use of FPPE may also be in follow-up to questions of care as a result of the OPPE process.

Specific highlights of the FPPE requirement for the medical staff process are that (1) the policy is universally applied regardless of background or training, (2) triggers and evaluative criteria have been developed a priori, (3) only specific privileges be reviewed, (4) a period of review be defined, and (5) actions to resolve performance gaps are clearly defined and consistently implemented. The information for the FPPE "may include chart review, monitoring clinical practice patterns, simulation, proctoring, external peer review, and discussion with other individuals involved in the care of each patient".[2] These sources are also used for OPPE.

The OPPE "allows the organization to identify professional practice trends that impact on quality of care and patient safety".[2] The sources for criteria may be "review of operative and other clinical procedures…, pattern of blood and pharmaceutical usage, requests of tests and procedures, LOS patterns, M&M data, use of consultants, and other relevant criteria as determined by the organized medical staff." The OPPE requirements are somewhat different from the FPPE: (1) there is a clearly defined process, (2) the type of data can be determined by departments, and (3) the information from the OPPE must be used in the determination of continuing, limiting, or revoking existing privileges.

Ironically, the basis for peer review in most hospitals is now due to TJC requirement—connecting peer review with the request and maintenance of

privilege of practice. Whether peer review would be completed on an organizational level without this requirement is unclear. And to extend this haziness, it is
unclear whether the form of "reviewing the practice of peers" would (or will) have
evolved beyond what is now compliance with TJC requirements. After observing
this culture for years, and typical of organizational behavior, once a compliance
threshold has been established most organizations provide minimally beyond
this mark (Figure 2-1). This is probably due to the lack of effective organizational
vision and leadership and the resulting lack of linkage between peer review, performance improvement, and strategic positioning within a competitive market-
place with patient betterment as a goal. Still, some sites have experimented with
modifications of the peer review process.[3]

TJC process is minimally about quality improvement and much more about
quality control. TJC does not promote a requirement to raise quality beyond
addressing performance where a gap has been observed. TJC could do more, promoting the concept of increasing performance as a goal; instead, TJC promotes
a policing concept as the FPPE is a gatekeeping mechanism and the OPPE (with
subsequent FPPE) works to identify outliers for mediation (revising or revoking
privileges). As per TJC blog by Robert Wise, MD,[4] "it is important to emphasize
that OPPE is not designed to identify clinicians who are delivering good or excellent
care." In fact, he identifies how the policy, based on implementation, could result in
negative outcomes, "the criteria used for OPPE may also identify some clinicians
who have no quality of care issues (ie, identification of situations that turn out to be
false positives)." This latter comment exposes the peer review policy as a disservice
to physicians—the idea that insufficient compliance with some local, potentially
non-EB standard or culture could result in being identified as an outlier. These physicians may actually practice beyond the state of the art, potentially better than the
local standard of care, and whose practice should be viewed positively! This policy
evokes the cultural issues within medical care that plague the evolution or innovation of practice. The system is set up to punish or reduce practice from objectivity
and improvement to protectiveness and though the outcome may not be specified
in the wording of TJC policy, the medical staff often interprets the policy as an effort
to remove nonstandard practice without determination of whether it is evidence
based. Indeed, within the policy there is no mention of "evidence-based" practice.

Despite its wording, current implementation, and functioning, within TJC
OPPE/FPPE policy structure is opportunity. As mentioned above, TJC allows for
compliance *and* opportunity for institutions/medical staff to develop more robust
approaches to physician performance including a cultural aspect of continuous
physician improvement and a forward vision of innovation. It is allowed and
up to the medical staff at the institution to require more of its physicians, not

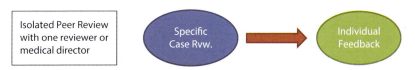

FIGURE 2-1. Methods of peer review—basic method.

as a method of control but as an organizational commitment to the betterment of practice by physicians for patients. Indeed the medical staff could take larger application steps beyond quality control[3]; one method would be committing to an auditing system described in Chapter 3 of this text.

■ COMMON DEPARTMENTAL STRUCTURE AND PROCESS

This section will describe the most common method of peer review: the retrospective chart review. As per Edwards and Benjamin, hospitals include many actions in a wide scope of activity under the heading of "peer review" but almost all continue to use the chart review as a fundamental activity to inspect care.[1] This section could be used to compare the reader's current practice review method, potentially to gain in new techniques or insights for the respective program.

Most departments or groups have a peer reviewer either the medical director or a designated physician(s). Notably, most organizations understand and have policy (written or unwritten) that the peer reviewer is not the physician associated with the case. Often, due to the supposedly noxious job that peer review is regarded as in many sites, several physicians perform the reviewing role annually and/or rotate responsibilities during the year or for a period. The hours for a review may be reimbursed or not. Interestingly, most physicians have no training in reviewing charts and this result is probably based on (1) the assumption of standard of care such that the reviewer has a "rubber stamp" mind-set and is just fulfilling a hospital requirement; (2) the chronic physician cultural resistance of review necessity; and (3) the lack of formal training related to nonclinical practice (though most would acknowledge that chart review has the potential to impact clinical practice!). See Figures 2-1 and 2-2.

Other organizations have defined committees for peer review and are usually hospital or organizationally based and not specialty specific or departmental (Figure 2-3). These committees could be composed of many different specialties such as obstetrics/gynecology, general or surgical specialties, anesthesia, etc, and though they fulfill a regulatory and possibly a risk-management responsibility, due to the lack of expertise in most of the cases they are of inconsistent

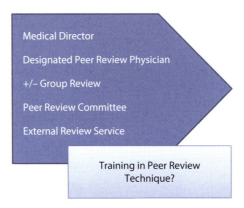

Medical Director

Designated Peer Review Physician

+/– Group Review

Peer Review Committee

External Review Service

Training in Peer Review Technique?

FIGURE 2-2. Reviewers in peer review.

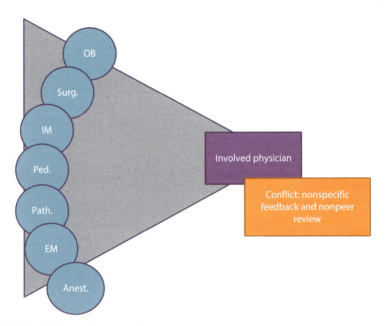

FIGURE 2-3. Peer review committee.

effectiveness in providing specific evidence-based feedback. Most of the time, these multispecialty committees have one or two specialty representatives (often medical directors) who attempt to explain the case to nonspecialty members. This is a poor mechanism as methods, goals, and specific literature vary per specialty and this kind of review is only "peer" in the broadest sense—a group of physicians. As an example, I mediated a multispecialty peer review committee's review of the management of a sepsis patient. Unfortunately, the committee was not accurate (probably due to the lack of specialty knowledge) enough in its criticism and resulted in a response letter:

> According to the letter's paragraph, "the Committee's decision is based on the lactate being ordered five hours after the patient was admitted to the hospital and two hours prior to his discharge [transfer]. If the lactate was ordered sooner it would have led to an earlier diagnosis of sepsis and to the appropriate hospital bed being ordered."
>
> I am concerned about the Committee's statement "if the lactate was ordered sooner it would have led to an earlier diagnosis of sepsis..." It is well stated in the above article[5] and is common knowledge in practice that physicians not use lactate to determine the diagnosis of sepsis. As per the original River's article the lactate was used to determine the need for ongoing resuscitation. Currently there is no marker that has been found to consistently confirm or refute the diagnosis of sepsis but many markers are actionable. Even 50% of blood cultures have no growth in patients thought to be septic. In this patient's case the lactate was completed during the resuscitation and was appropriately

used to continue aggressive measures. Studies support that a persistently ele-
vated lactate results in an increased patient mortality but this is a marker for
continued resuscitation not a marker confirming diagnosis. Conversely and
inappropriately I have seen physicians using a negative lactate as grounds to
discharge patients or to ignore further treatment of infection. Certainly by
the Committee's inference, the Committee is not advocating this latter role
for serum lactate as it is not evidence-based medicine? I would appreciate a
response with this clarification and reassurance of this organization's commit-
ment to evidence-based medicine.

Getting past the sarcasm, hopefully everyone was more knowledgeable after
the interaction.

Like all review systems, current peer review is dependent on the mechanism
of entering cases into review; in the case of emergency medicine, most systems
have entry points for chart review from simple referrals by other physicians to set
triggers such as return visits within 72 hours and all mortalities associated with
the emergency department (Figure 2-4).[1] Other triggers could be incident reports,
referrals from medical staff committees, members or hospital departments, complication reports, readmission reports, and patient /family complaints (issues of
clinical quality not satisfaction). One study observed the use of Rapid Response
Team events within 24 hours of ED admission as entry data.[6]

Using the preset triggers, cases are identified through the medical staff or
quality improvement offices at the hospital and forwarded to the reviewing
physician(s). Usually routine peer review is delayed for several weeks from time
of care due to the steps in the process, in the identification of patients, and often
due to the activity as a nonpriority for the physicians involved (see culture statement above). The irregularity in the process flow could be compounded with
patient satisfaction cases and risk management cases entered into the "pipeline"
for review (single reviewer) depending on the job duties and need of expeditious

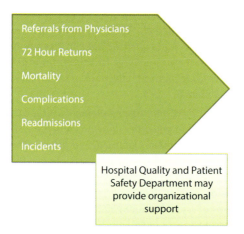

FIGURE 2-4. Generic triggers for chart identification in peer review.

review. Many departments separate patient complaints (billing and service questions) from clinical review due to the volume of work and probably the necessity of the medical director to be involved in the former. Understandably, there should be some communication or linkage between those reviewers as this could provide a more robust program of physician feedback. Considering the potential for "burnout" in emergency physicians, an awareness of an increasing frequency of case events in both the patient satisfaction and clinical realm could lead to earlier physician intervention and career mediation.

Some organizations, potentially with more enlightened visions of quality improvement, have added criteria to include system issues within peer review. This I applaud as (1) it is a rare event that allows a review of physician performance in a vacuum, the exception is in the setting of a procedure in which a technique error can receive 100% attribution to the physician, and (2) the modern concept of complex organizational error is the "Swiss cheese" model in which many microerrors or events align in sequence to result in a major negative outcome. One example, included below in the case studies, of system or operational challenges is in the case of *Patient X- MRN 1124438* in which the lack of equipment (lack of GlidoScope covers and IO equipment within the ED) was involved in the management of the case, and had a potential to contribute to the outcome as well as the potential to compromise future patient care. As important as providing feedback to the physician involved in the case, a well-defined process for addressing identifiable system issues within the peer review process must be functional, assignable, and provide loop closure. Also included below is a summary from another case (a root cause analysis) of key actions and assignments in order to track responsibility for process change.

Few groups ask the reviewer to base critique on pertinent articles in the literature (Figure 2-5). Physicians should always attempt to remain objective within peer criticism (several challenges were mentioned above), relating the case to specific literature, preferably peer reviewed. When the review is based on literature, the physician has the opportunity to receive a conclusion with less resistance, due to the presumed objectivity of the literature. This allows for more openness to consider practice change.

Sometimes in "smaller, closer" families (small physician groups, usually not emergency physician groups), the need for external review to maintain harmony and objectivity is required. Consider a three-physician neurosurgical group, even though neurosurgeons are superhuman (humor), and can remain perfectly objective within their own cases (humor), this group should request outside sources for formal peer review.

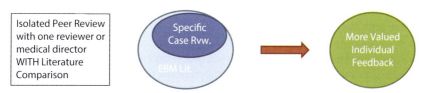

FIGURE 2-5. Methods of peer review—use of evidence-based literature.

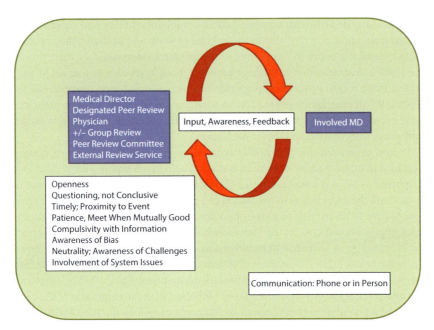

FIGURE 2-6. Reviewer and involved physician interaction.

Peer review should never be completed without the input from the physician reviewed (Figure 2-6). This is just poor form and represents a punitive culture lacking in transparency and in the vision of improving care. A medical director or reviewer can never be so busy or the issue so conclusive that communication about the case with the involved physician is unnecessary. If the goal is learning and practice change then a humanistic, interactive process must be established and supported. Certainly, the potential for conflict and argument in a discussion is present with the outreach but so is the amazing opportunity for collegiality and raising practice to a higher level of quality. It is about communication technique.

It has been my experience that with the notification of a review the involved physician automatically and immediately responds with some surface resistance but also applies a self-critical and negative interpretation of his/her of care. The earlier notification the better as the involved physician will have a better memory and response of a proximate case to an older case. The job of the reviewer (which is the reason for training in this role) is to initiate the conversation with an openness of language and a willingness to listen (suspended judgment). It is critical that the involved physician not feel "blindsided" and is given opportunity to share. Often with sharing he or she will move through various layers of response from defensive to introspective. To enable this process, the reviewer should contact the involved physician by phone or in person (not e-mail and certainly not by a standardized formal letter!) and confirm an appropriate time to talk. Usually allowing one or more days to pass after notification will remove some angst and resistance about the review. Choosing a good time and a neutral place—not after a night shift (tired) and not before a shift (rushed and not what he/she should be thinking

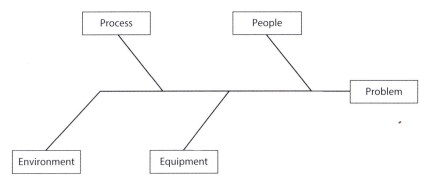

FIGURE 2-7. System issues represented by fishbone diagram incorporated into peer review.

about during a current shift)—allowing the involved physician some determination of course is helpful. Be patient and make the feedback process convenient for the involved physician not necessarily for you.

Moreover, much is often unwritten within the chart such that the whole story surrounding the case is not present for the reviewer. This is especially apparent within the emergency department in which system issues often impact the physician and the environment or setting of the case (Figure 2-7).[7] One obvious example is reviewing the pattern of shifts of the involved physician prior to the day of the reviewed case with the understanding that exhaustion is a negative factor in performance. Other examples are volume stress within the department due to crowding (well known to cause gaps in care and compromised outcomes)[8] or nursing shortages and misalignment of ability with the higher acuity of presenting patient.[9]

Recently, I was able to observe a terrible display of feedback. The incoming EM physician had barely set down his bag and logged into the work computer to start his shift when the ED nurse manager approached him about a prior patient's outcome. The physician spent the next 45 minutes reviewing the chart, speaking again with the ED nurse manager, and informally "defending" his care with the other two physicians (myself and another) who were present and had overheard the "information." Several points on this event can be observed. First, the physician did not initiate any new care for the first 45 minutes of his shift when there were patients waiting to be seen, thus he was not able to fulfill his primary role and focus during a critical transition time in the department. Second, this distracting feedback was not presented at a time or place adequate for learning but caused the physician to respond defensively. Despite his effort to focus, very few physicians would have the ability to limit the ongoing consideration of the case and thus this issue will remain in his consciousness throughout the remaining period and potentially compromise his current evaluations and efficiency. Third, the ED nurse manager was inappropriate to act in this way as she did not have a formal role in physician case review and, ironically, her own actions compromised ED flow and patient throughput. (I suspect a bit of a power play [wink]).

Getting back to the conversation between the physician reviewer and the physician involved in the case, it is important that the reviewer present the absolute "challenges" of the case initially, again affirming that medicine is difficult. One technique, especially valuable, is a method of asking questions for clarification. Comparatively, conclusive statements do not move the process forward well, and threats or ultimatums are not educational or found to be successful in creating higher functioning and sustained change.

In my years of performing and participating in peer review, I have concluded that one can tell the quality of practice and the depth, supportiveness, and well-being of the group by exploring the review process within it. The method of review represents the culture of the group. It can be policing and managed by a single medical director anxious about control or due to the disinterest of the physician group. Conversely it can be collegial and open, allowing for education and supports group development. Many programs are positioned somewhere in the middle and hopefully this text can assist in the evolution of your review process. Interestingly, the group's peer review process does not have to have alignment with the contract structure between physicians and the organization though it often follows. I have seen independent contractor "groups" with consistent, established review programs and I have seen private practice groups with nonsupporting programs, though groups with less migration of physicians tend to have more developed reviewing methods (and often better culture).

■ THE ART OF THE PEER REVIEWER

As a peer reviewer, it is necessary to place oneself in two different but simultaneous positions: (1) evoking a sympathetic vision of the error-prone physician and an awareness of the decision-making steps that may have caused the event due to the fact that practicing medicine is extremely difficult[10] and *equally important*, (2) being the aggressive advocate or representative for the patient and having a zealous, "never again" mind-set to the process in order to avoid future similar conflicts (Figure 2-8).

As much as there is really no formal training for peer review; the physician reviewer has limited structure to follow.[11,12] Over the years I have developed a series of questions/points as a framework to help organize the review. Consider these general categories below (Figure 2-9):

- Preparation: Obtain all records about the case—include nursing notes, triage records, pertinent past visits, subsequent admission records, imaging interpretations.
- Read through the case several times making notes in the margins of the printout. Protect the documents—this is HIPAA!

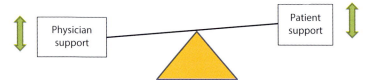

FIGURE 2-8. The art of the peer reviewer—a difficult balance.

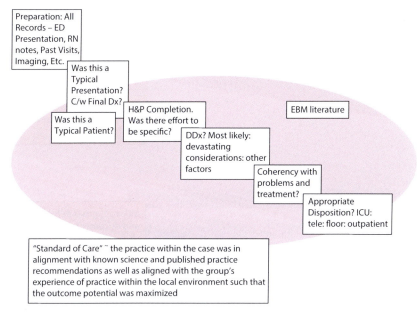

FIGURE 2-9. The peer review process—single case steps for review and/or preparation for group presentation.

- Replacing oneself as the practicing physician (attempting to be "everyman" or an equivalent actor) allows for better consideration of the case:
  - Is the presentation typical of the final diagnosis? (How do *I* feel [simulating] walking into the patient's room knowing the chief complaint?)
  - Is this a typical patient? Is the complaint typical of the patient type? What is common is common; the diabetic has a more likely chance of infection; the patient with CHF in the past has the potential to be in heart failure when he/she presents with SOB.
  - Was the H&P complete? Would others have asked more questions or fewer? Was the patient in such duress that adequate history was not possible at the time? Were other sources identified and used? Was the examination specific to the patient? (The basic concept I subscribe to in these reviews is that if any physician makes effort to understand the patient then it should be notable in the record and, historically, often results in successful outcomes and interactions.) *Soapbox*: This is one current problem with high volume "mills" that I have witnessed; these EDs or "mills" are blandly testing and treating patients without evidence of distinguishing patients (eg, 20 year old with CP vs 55 year old with CP—both get the same cocktail of testing and treatment). Frighteningly the physicians' records (often templates) show no uniqueness or distinctness to the presentation and one concludes that there was an utter lack of thoughtfulness to the exchange (Figure 2-10).

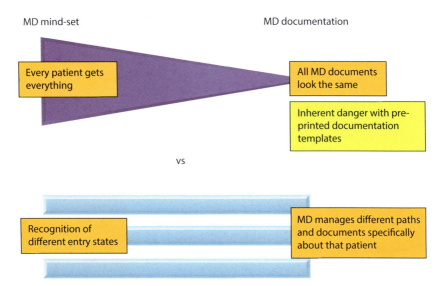

FIGURE 2-10. Reviewing a record and an interpretation of the MD mind-set.

- Was a differential diagnosis created?
  - This is a key component of the review as the differential diagnosis within the MDM supports the actions taken (this is the thinking physician).
  - Often I break a differential diagnosis into components (developed while teaching residents). Did the physician (1) identify the most obvious or likely problems; (2) consider the symptoms could represent a devastating process within our specialty focus (MI, PE, perforated bowel, sepsis, airway compromise, etc); (3) identify other factors, social or environmental, may complicate this presentation and subsequent management (language barriers, etc)? See Table 2-2.
- Was the treatment typical of the problems and the working diagnosis (coherency)? Were all problems adequately explained or addressed? Was the physician's response to the problems typical of what other physicians would do? What would I have done? (This cannot be the only factor but is important). What would others in my group have done? (This is where the group process [below] removes all guesswork.)
- Was the disposition appropriate? If admitted, floor or ICU? If discharged, was follow-up documented well and consistent with the problems as well as the combination of problems presented (a combination of the levels of the DDx as mentioned above has the potential to complicate disposition).

Within all of the subjective consideration must be implanted the objectivity of the literature. *In every reviewed case, the physician reviewer must be highly cautious of his/her own knowledge.* It is not beneficial to state one's own practice as a standard. *The best approach is to question even those items that one internally agrees*

■ TABLE 2-2. Framework for Differential Diagnosis	
Identify the most obvious or likely problems	42-year-old hypertensive, smoker with pleuritic CP probably has pleurisy
Consider the symptoms could represent a devastating process	But he could have acute coronary syndrome, aortic dissection, pulmonary embolus, pneumothorax, etc
Identify other factors, social or environmental, may complicate this presentation and subsequent management	He continues to smoke and has not taken his blood pressure medication for several months due to job loss and no income

with as well as the items that one has concerns over and methodically review the literature to confirm or refute each position or fact. Thus the peer review is an attempt to vigorously review the reviewer's knowledge as well as the involved physician's practice (which if done well causes the reviewer to heighten his/her practice also!).

Fortunately, the reviewer has the outcome or result and the necessary time to review that the involved physician did not. Still, the reviewer also has to be cautious about knowing the result of the case and the inherent bias with knowing the outcome. Outcomes also vary: a pneumothorax from a central-line placement is straightforward (but does this mean technique was bad?), whereas a death from community-acquired pneumonia not obvious (abnormal CXR but not indicative of infiltrate) on presentation is less. A comprehensive review is required including many factors in order to assist in feedback.

Finally, the overall philosophy of the reviewer (which also should extend to the group environment if the group reviews cases) is that physicians are fallible but malleable human beings and the practice of medicine is immensely challenging.[10] Was there compulsivity yet still an unexpected outcome? Sometimes despite best efforts, progression of disease occurs. Peer review should only be a learning event.

I rarely use the term, "standard of care" throughout most of this process description or when I review and/or lead a group discussion. I would rather have the goal in the case comparison as "the practice within the case was in alignment with known science and published practice recommendations as well as aligned with the group's experience of practice within the local environment such that the outcome potential was maximized" (Figure 2-11).

Some discrepancies in the review are less associated with the outcomes than others. Consider the review included a choice of antibiotic that is not first line but not inappropriate either according to the literature sources; allowance of this variation is acceptable. The objectives of peer review must be performance improvement as well as quality control. If the goal of peer review is also about performance improvement, the reviewer and the group must press each other further and look to each case as opportunities of improvement and the betterment of practice. This is when the group process is immensely helpful (if done well); providing some

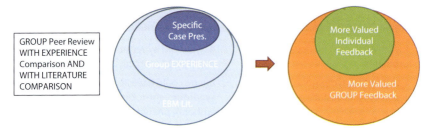

FIGURE 2-11. Methods of peer review—comprehensive peer review including group feedback and learning.

review literature or the microbiology patterns for the hospital during the discussion of the above case example allows for a discussion on these antibiotic choices.

After the review, the reviewing physician or the medical director should provide feedback to the physician involved in the care, usually in a one-on-one verbal manner and often in written form as well as a record of compliance with TJC requirements but also if the department or group has a robust tracking system for events (Figure 2-12). Alternatively or in conjunction with the individual feedback, groups will have cases presented and discussed during the monthly group/department meeting with either the group determining the adequacy of care or having a more general, learning discussion about the case and not attempting to judge the care. Some groups attempt to be anonymous in the case presentation using the reviewer or the medical director as the presenter. Often the involved physician participates in the group review and discussion. Thus it is especially important to inform the involved physician well ahead of the review and/or the presentation of the case, though not necessarily for him or her to gather a defense but as mentioned earlier to reduce the initial resistance to practice review and give time

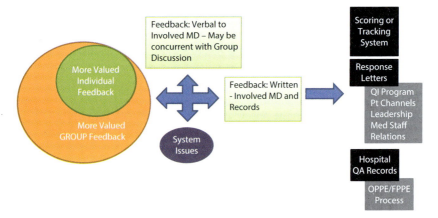

FIGURE 2-12. Comprehensive feedback process with peer review.

to develop an openness for introspection. This then allows him/her to absorb colleagues' thoughts on the case.

Group discussion has advantage over one-on-one discourse as the group presentations allow for information transfer and the discussion could lead to heightened practice awareness within the group.[10,13] This is especially important in emergency medicine as group members often practice alone during a shift, which limits knowledge sharing. The intermittent presence within the department also limits collective knowledge distribution or translation (Figure 2-13).

During a group review, when the director or the reviewer makes effort to review the foundational literature on the case, he/she potentially allows each physician participant, not just the physician associated with the case, to compare his/her experience with evidence-based literature. This concept of peer review, a blending of data-directed behavior and experience (personal stories of cases and outliers) (Figure 2-11), could enable a robust conversation within the meeting about local clinical practice and national patterns and overall heighten the potential for a modification of practice quality throughout the physician group. One roll of the physician reviewer and presenter is to provide the national pattern as interpreted through the literature. Again, mechanistically, this achieves the concept of standard of care defined previously as the combination of experience and evidence.

Below is an explanation and outline I provide to the presenters of cases for group peer review processes (amended for space):

1. *Case presentation (5-10 minutes)—timeline and circumstance—allowance for questions for clarification—no discussion at this time.*

2. *Literature presentation/Review (20-30 minutes)—based on literature search and chapter review— I would pick out interesting points or topics that you did not remember and when you read them a light bulb went on saying "ah! I knew this once" or "hey that is helpful" plus I think it is good to do some general review—go over the basics of clinical presentation and approach; differential*

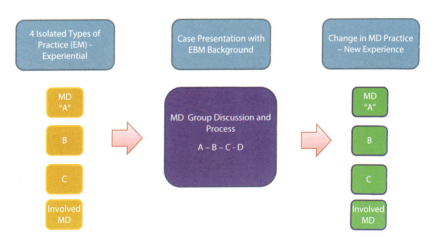

FIGURE 2-13. Impact on physician practice—the value of group discussion.

diagnosis; and any procedure that might go with the topic. We will try to stay "evidence based" if there is good evidence. Should be minimal interruptions during this— no discussion at this time— just run through the presentation.

Example:

Topic: Pediatric Altered MS (general)

Topic: Ventricular Shunts and complications (specific)

For Change in MS:

> *Pediatric presentation*
>
> *Approach to this—differential dx*

For VPS:

> *Pediatric presentation—challenges*
>
> *Complications—specifics*
>
> *Obstruction—types*

Summary: Fine points of presentation

Take home points to keep us sharp, improved, and risk free

3. *Time for limited discussion (5-10 minutes) of case based on presentation.*
4. *Format can either be simple paper handout outline (one page) or PowerPoint presentation.*

Note that most of the group discussions are rarely if ever contained to 10 minutes! But clearly the goal of the blending of the literature with experience and providing a format for both sections is a helpful structure.

Unfortunately, peer review is rarely the affirmation of practice; usually a most positive conclusion of a review is that practice was adequate and opportunity for improvement was not present. Again this fits the compliance and quality control model and is the basis of criticism about peer review—largely that the physician feels like he or she has "dodged a bullet," wasted time, and really practice has not improved (Figure 2-14). Peer reviewers should approach cases looking for opportunities for affirming good care despite the potential in the process structure to focus only on the negatives.[10]

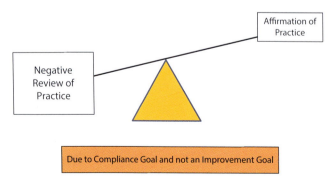

FIGURE 2-14. The imbalance of practice support with results of standard peer review.

It is also important to publicly acknowledge successful practice, affirming behaviors that increase patient safety and outcomes. Indeed, Edwards and Benjamin[1] noted that only 6% of hospitals recognized clinicians for excellent performance. Despite this infrequency, remarkable affirmation of care can occur during group review due to and supporting a stronger cultural cohesiveness within the department.

Croskerry[7] discusses the concept of calibration as the "accuracy of an individual's probability assessments" with both positive and negative feedback allowing continued calibration of clinical judgment. As mentioned above if the departmental peer review is a group process, all participants have the opportunity to undergo recalibration. Peer review does not have to be about bad outcomes if the goal is about raising a group's quality of practice. A restructuring the review process is all that is necessary. Indeed, some organizations are attempting this.[1] One of the distinct differences between standard peer review and a clinical auditing program such as the SCA described in Chapter 3 is that the SCA structure exposes and affirms higher valued or quality care while also fulfilling the basic peer review functioning.

Some departments or peer review committees construct a scoring or grading system as an attempt to provide more objectivity to the review. The grading is coarse and usually involves three or more categories. Usually these scoring systems are not complex enough to be predictive, thus they should be cautiously used if at all in connection with privileges or other medical staff or physician group activity or governance. Clearly this is an attempt to objectify the process with the understanding that tracking single events could present trends and that looking at error "loads" over time may add meaning to the process. The goal is an attempt to use the data in a patient safety emphasis for more assistance than credentialing. Adding to the complexity of the peer review process acknowledges the complexity of practice.

Below is a grading system that we proposed for one group:

Addendum 1 [Practice Monitoring]:

Institute a value system or significance level to further define the practice error.

Creating a numeric system assigned a significance level creates a universal structure under which all sites can objectively rate an error as well as aids monitoring and standardizes the subsequent referral to the Quality Committee due significance, trends, or volume over time

An error in judgment on choosing which test to study a child's abdominal pain resulting in inconclusive data and leading to another test or delay in care has not the significance as a decision to discharge a 50-year-old with active CP and a history of angina. Both are errors of practice, yet one has catastrophic implications, not just delay in care. A significant level or value should be employed with each categorization of error. A significance level of "1" or SL1 could mean a single issue or error, isolated and not catastrophic; a "SL2" is associated with multiple or complex errors or issues, or generally poor management/judgment on many aspects of the case, but not catastrophic; and a "SL3" is a catastrophic or opportunity for such (implication in the demise of the patient) error. The SL could be associated with each error. For example— an error in suturing resulting in wound dehiscence (SL1) vs an error in central-line placement resulting in PTX (SL3); both are errors in technique (Table 2-3). The same case could have an error in judgment that could also be rated according to significance level.

Based on the above (2) discussion on valuing the error, it is important to recognize that distinct events should be reviewed as well as trends in care. Referral triggers could be (1) any SL3 event and (2) a volume or sum of SL errors over time. The latter system could be a summation of the SL1—three errors reflecting a trend in practice. A threshold could be 10 SL "points" in 6 months and 15 SL "points" in 12 months. Again this is a proposal; the numbers mentioned here are estimates to provide a justified trigger being as least stringent but responsive, functional, and objective. Example of the system would be a physician who over the course of 6 months has an SL3, two SL2s, and three SL1s; would trigger the committee to initiate a formal review of the MDs practice. This does not preclude the request of the medical director from a site, the president, or the medical staff to request a review of the practice of an MD or to review an event that has significant impact on the whole group (risk management, behavioral, interdepartmental [affecting status within the hospital]). Tracking this system requires the peer reviewers from each site to maintain a file of all cases requiring "opportunity for improvement" in order to track SL errors, and a form need be created to document the "second tier" review and its findings. This form should summarize the event, provide error descriptions, document actions and decisions taken by the QI committee, and have area to report follow-up/feedback. The president and the site Medical Director should be informed of the findings.

Interestingly, we developed and managed a scoring or tracking system at one site and were able to identify a pattern of significant clinical events for one

TABLE 2-3. A Scoring or Grading System for Peer Review Events

Significance Level	Definition	Example
SL1	Single issue; isolated; noncatastrophic	Suture dehiscence
SL2	Multiple or series of SL1s, or complex case but not catastrophic	Suture dehiscence with *no* documentation or consideration of FB; questionable technique
SL3	Catastrophic event or the potential for catastrophe	Wire left in chest or vascular system from CVC insertion and no CXR obtained

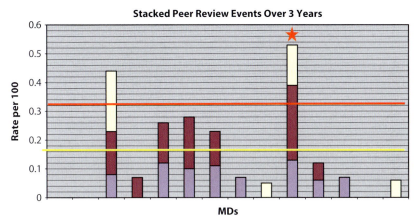

FIGURE 2-15. Tracking peer review events per physician (one group). (Colors represent different years; yellow horizontal line—mean; red—1 SD; star represents physician intervention; 3 MDs without any review.)

physician in comparison to the group (Figure 2-15). Many of the cases had a high significance level though we had not employed that grading in the group. Our engagement with that physician allowed the recognition of multiple external, personal factors impacting his/her clinical quality and focus. Intervention ensued.

In addition to feedback to the involved physician as above, "closing the loop" of peer review supports many goals of an organization though time consuming (Table 2-4). A response letter for a referral or a summary for a triggered chart review is essential for communication. Writing a letter responding to complaints about patient care is important for several business and political reasons: an

■ TABLE 2-4. "Closing the Loop" in the Peer Review Process

Arena	Specifics
Clinical practice change	Individual feedback
	Group process feedback
Political	Improving group culture
	Marketing practice value to administration
	Medical staff relations
	Institutional leadership
Business	Supporting patient channels
Memory	Group or medical director records and coordination of practice quality
	Hospital TJC compliance

indication or advertisement that the group wants to improve and has a process for this (always good that hospital administration knows); taking a nonspecialty colleague's concerns seriously (medical staff relations); clearly a business sense of encouraging patient channels (contract and financials); and finally trying to evoke a culture of continuous performance improvement and patience (leadership) within the institution. The hospital should be keeping records of the reviews in order to confirm compliance with TJC OPPE/FPPE requirements, though sometimes this is a simple form indicating completion. The peer reviewer should keep case review records in the event that questions occur in the future about a colleague's care, if peer review is embedded within a larger quality improvement program, or if the reviewer chooses in the future to write a book about physician performance (hmmm). Of course, all records must be HIPAA compliant.

What is the outcome of current peer review? Within some physician groups (whether stated explicitly or not), the goal is individual or group education and resultant modification of practice for improved care and outcomes, though, as mentioned above, peer review in many sites is a compliance process. In reflection on OPPE/FPPE, it is my experience that rarely current peer review results in the dismissal of a physician (a revocation of all privileges). At most institutions I suspect that the TJC-compliant peer review process has been made anemic or passive since the process is not representative of overall practice, thus governing physicians, acknowledging this, limit outcome severity. Unfortunately, the local implementation of the OPPE and FPPE requirements could be modified to the level that few practice events trigger action and in that respect, inconsistent, non-EBM practice might avoid recognition. In the end, most organizations could do better, embedding the required peer review quality control process in a more aggressive, performance auditing process.[1,14]

Soapbox: A comment on a proposed concept of "self-reporting"—ideally in a nonpunitive culture that emphasizes continuous improvement in the policy of "raising one's hand and identifying one's responsibility in an error" is a healthy addition. Unfortunately, current culture and policy as per the above discussion limit support of this behavior. Depending on his or her judgment as to whether the peer review process is more policing or more practice improvement, a physician should choose whether to stick his or her proverbial "neck out" or not. As we will see in Chapter 3, clinical auditing removes this conflict with a process change (that could lead to cultural change) that results in the continuous, universal, transparent review of practice.

■ CASE STUDIES IN PEER REVIEW

The following are case reviews provided as nonidentifiable (HIPAA compliant) examples. Comments are inserted within the material in order to emphasize points of the above discussion. These cases were modified from various groups over many years and represent the complexity of medical care as well as the need for comprehensiveness when reviewing.

PATIENT X

Clinical Summary—Mortality

This is a peer review summary on the X case, based on a policy of reviewing of all mortalities within the X Emergency Department or occurring within 72 hours of admission from the ED.

There is value to identifying the trigger for the peer review. It helps physicians accept the universality and entry objectivity.

Mr X entered the ED with hypotension and abdominal pain; he further decompensated within the department and had a cardiac arrest with unsuccessful resuscitation. His autopsy identified mesenteric ischemia as the probable cause of his abdominal pain and death.

I have reviewed the case and prior two visits this patient had to the X ED. I have reviewed the autopsy report, spoken with staff involved in the patient's care and with the primary ED physician, Dr. X.

Below are bullets points on the factors identified that are conflicts/components to care and have association with the outcome. The method of bulleting these items helps provide structure to the participants/group as these are "digestible" points in the care and can be points of discussion or assignable for quality improvement of processes. Further, the flow of the report would be according to the time sequence of the case; thus the summary attempts to place the reviewer within the case and milestones helping him or her develop a similar mind-set of the involved physician.

Considerations:

- The patient's abnormal vital signs (VS) were identified on presentation and appropriate placement into a main ED resuscitation room occurred. Dr. X. recognized the abnormal VS and compared to prior emergency department visits.

Important to reference the records for factual support to the assessment of care—especially noting past visits that frame the current presentation and assist in understanding the individual patient status. It is important also to identify when processes have been well followed, a policy of obtaining VS on every patient.

There is some challenge in interpreting the patient's clinical status based on the abnormal values; this patient, with end-stage renal disease, had chronically low blood pressure and was on an outpatient regimen to maintain an adequate blood pressure. Distinct on this visit, the patient had persistent tachycardia; the heart rate either had been in a normal range or had normalized on past visits. The patient was chronically hypothermic on each of the last three ED visits.

- Dr. X. considered potential devastating illness on presentation. A CT scan of the abdomen was ordered early in the evaluation; oral contrast was ordered.

Dr. X. reports considering pain control but was concerned about causing a worsening in hypotension. This is a frequent challenge within the ED and a prudent response is often to withhold analgesia out of concern for decompensation.

- The above VS could be interpreted as shock or sepsis in this patient until proven otherwise, but the history of hypotension confuses the interpretation of VS. Again, Dr. X. and the staff recognized the potential instability. If the standard sepsis algorithm is considered, the patient had a chronically abnormal MAP and thus this value would not be clinically valuable. Thus a lactate level would benefit the early resuscitation course. The lactate was obtained with entry labs; results verbally reported 90 minutes later—this is probably adequate considering the first 6 hours of resuscitation for sepsis. According to the sepsis standards a lactate >4 with or without hypotension (MAP <65) requires ongoing resuscitation response.

Referring to EB literature provides objectivity to the review process; in this case, reference was to standard sepsis criteria well known to EM.

Crystalloid resuscitation should be aggressively initiated—it appears 1 L of NS was ordered and infused and 1 L NS was given by EMS. Volume (crystalloid and blood products) should be continued until lactate normalized, MAP >65, or CVP within normal range (8-12 mm Hg).

- Blood glucose by EMS was normal.
- One of the other challenges with this patient is the appreciation of the patient's volume status. The patient with end-stage renal disease can have intravascular depletion, pump failure, volume overload, or a combination of the three. Noted in the history, the patient had not obtained hemodialysis in the prior days; this would indicate potential volume overload. Although acute hypotension requires volume resuscitation, this clinical picture and response are very complex.
- No vasopressors were ordered until cardiac arrest occurred.
- This case appears to also have challenging IV access. A peripheral access was obtained by the ambulance service. PIV was also obtained by staff (R upper chest and RUE)—labs were obtained within 30 minutes of presentation. In reading the physician's note there appeared to be an attempt at obtaining larger venous access—internal jugular access was attempted by Drs. X. and Y. but was unsuccessful. Subsequent CXR showed no pneumothorax.
  - It is unclear whether this delayed or distracted ongoing resuscitation.
  - Ultrasound was utilized.
  - Subclavian venous access is noncompressible and the patient was coagulopathic. Dr. X. reported that he considered femoral venous access but deferred for placement of the IO due to the challenges with the IJ access at the time. A femoral CVC was placed during ACLS resuscitation.

- An IO was placed subsequently. The team should be commended for this approach. IO access can be a bridge in crisis and allow for adequate resuscitation. Unfortunately, the X ED IO tool and its parts could not be found; Dr. X. reports he had to request an EMS crew obtain the EMS IO equipment from the EMS vehicle. This is an inadequate response within the ED. Several considerations should be reviewed: the standardization of access, the training of IO placement, and staff knowledge of the storage site. These areas will be forwarded to ED leadership.

Noted system or process problem that will be referred to the leadership or management team. Usually a retrospective case review will have many system or process findings; see below for a list (different case) of process improvements.

- The first venous blood gas which showed significant acidosis—pH 7.02—and confirmed the concerns of the staff and provider. A subsequent blood gas showed improvement though a poorly compensated metabolic acidosis persisted— pH 7.31. Still this was reassuring that the resuscitation provided was improving the clinical position. A third blood gas pH 7.13 showed worsening acidosis.
- Rapid-sequence intubation per Dr. X. was complicated. Dr. X. reports requesting the GlidoScope but was informed that the covers were not accessible within the ED and this caused delay in intubation. Knowledge of the equipment and timely, consistent access is necessary. This process requires a review and will be forwarded to the ED leadership. Unfortunately, there is variation per physician on methods of airway control which has the potential to complicate the ED activity and may frequently challenge the staff. A thorough review of the resuscitation equipment within each resuscitation room may be necessary.

Noted system or process problem that will be referred to the leadership or management team.

- It is unclear what caused the rapid cardiovascular decompensation immediately after intubation. There was no pneumothorax. The patient was known to have CAD and with hypotension myocardial ischemia could have occurred. Severe acidosis could have contributed to cardiac arrest as well. The medications for RSI were standard agents.
- Because this was a complex patient and presentation, there appeared to be several calls and consultations during the resuscitation. These are a challenge to balance: remaining at bedside with minute to minute management versus the necessity of involving specialists in the care of this complex, clinically unstable patient. Often phone calls require the provider to leave the bedside. A review of the methods and consistency of communication within the department is suggested.

Noted system or process problem that will be referred to the leadership or management team.

- The patient's blood work showed a significant drop in the patient's hemoglobin. On a prior visit the HGB was 14 and this had decreased to 9 on presentation. Early blood product resuscitation was considered. An order for FFP infusion and an order for PRBCs transfusion were given. The patient was coagulopathic with an INR of 9; he received vitamin K 5 mg IV as well as the above product. Dr. X. reports some confusion with communicating the need for blood products, and specifically attributes this to the complexity of steps required to order blood products through CPOE. Confirmation of this problem will occur with direct inquiry to other providers and a subsequent IT review as indicated.
- Considering the antibiotic choice, both Vancomycin and Zosyn were provided and dosages were standard and appropriate. The addition of Flagyl would be reasonable though it is unlikely this would change the outcome. It appears by dictation that with the recognition of the elevated white blood cell count, antibiotics were initiated. The antibiotics were ordered within the recommended sepsis guideline of 3 hours. Blood cultures were obtained prior to antibiotic infusion and do not appear to have delayed therapy initiation.

Referring to EB literature provides objectivity to the process; in this case, reference was to standard sepsis criteria well known to EM.

- There appeared to be early surgical consultation, but this was focused on the AV graft with a comment in Dr. X's note that the abdomen was assessed. In Dr. X's dictation, Dr. Z. was also consulted by phone and recommended CT scan prior to his bedside evaluation.
- There was also early consultation with the ICU team. This appears to be a case in which early, joint management would be valuable. Discussion with the ICU leadership should occur on this concept. Further, the author and Dr. X. in conversation reflected on the options to delay CT scanning and transfer this patient earlier to the ICU for ongoing resuscitation. This method of management, the prioritizing of stabilization prior to specific diagnosis by imaging, was used in the past and may have value in some resuscitation events. Further discussion on this management method should occur between services.
- Dr. X. reports adequate numbers of ED staff support.
- Autopsy: acute GI bleeding; small bowel and ascending colon necrosis and thinning. Clinical note on mesenteric ischemia and ESRD: hypotension is a known cause of mesenteric ischemia and this patient potentially had chronic low flow to the mesentery. A further reduction in the blood pressure could result in ischemia and infarction of bowel and this probably occurred prior to the ED presentation.

Summary of potential improvements:
- Ongoing review sepsis bundle goals with X providers and staff. Dr. X. was challenged with the clinical presentation but achieved many the elements of the

sepsis bundle including early lactate, volume resuscitation, antibiotics. Early vasopressor treatment could be recommended.

- ED IO process and access needs review.
- ED GlidoScope process needs review.
- ED communication needs ongoing development and review.
- Review CVC methods of access with all X providers.
- Review IT CPOE process for blood product ordering for accuracy and efficiency.
- Discuss with ED leadership value of dialogue with ICU team and leadership on joint resuscitation concept.
- Final note: The staff and provider response to the critically ill in the department has unique challenges requiring heightened communication and teamwork, heightened clinical skills, and the support of ED processes. When expected efficiency and/or even overall success are not achieved, often the personal stress of participating in the uncontrolled situation becomes evident during the resuscitation and afterward. Provider and staff styles vary and should be acceptable within limits but processes should be standard and consistent and not become a component of the resuscitation team stress. Instead, ED processes should be to such a state as to reduce the stress within the event. Further work needs be completed within the X ED to ensure consistency in response to maximize team resuscitation, interaction, and mutual support.

PATIENT Y

Clinical Summary—Mortality

This is a peer review summary on the Patient X case. Patient X presented to the ED with the chief complaint of weakness. EMS report noted a fall and weakness. The patient was evaluated in the ED, had a LOS >5 hours; and decompensated during the ED evaluation resulting in intubation. The CT imaging identified an ICH and the patient was determined to be coagulopathic possibly due to poor compliance with primary care physician recommendations (please see Dr. X's addendum record). The patient underwent craniotomy with Dr. Y. Postoperatively the patient continued to have unresolving neurological compromise and died.

I have reviewed the documentation associated with the ED management and reviewed a peer review document per Ms A. I have spoken with Dr. X.

Important to reference the records for factual support to the assessment of care—especially noting past visits that frame the current presentation and assist in understanding the individual patient status. It is valuable to note the sources of information for the report, especially affirming to all physicians is the conversation with the involved physician and not an isolated review of charting.

Considerations:

- EMS report noted complaints of altered MS and fall. Combined with the knowledge that the patient was on Coumadin and could be interpreted as high risk for ICH.

- EMS report provided a list of medications—including Coumadin—that contrasted to the medication list of the primary assessment. It appears that the primary assessment medication list is associated with a prior visit and not updated with the EMS list and current visit. This appears conflicting with the medication reconciliation process or goal and with this specific case could lead to significant medical error. Fortunately, Dr. X. noted the medications on interviewing the patient and identified the use of Coumadin by the patient.

  Noted system or process problem that will be referred to the leadership or management team.

- Recheck of blood sugar—EMS identified hypoglycemia requiring treatment and triage recorded this action. One of the initial interventions on a patient who received treatment for hypoglycemia would be to recheck the blood sugar level. There is no evidence that this recheck occurred in the ED until the serum chemistry was resulted with a normal serum glucose hours after entry.

- Dr. X. evaluated the patient initially—noting concern for fall, altered MS, and Coumadin use. Dr. X. initiated the CT order. No INR level was provided at time of Dr. X's initial evaluation.

- Operationally, the ED volume was 30 patients above average—Please see the attached peer review note with the "ED Staffing" for staffing levels. In regard to the ED volume and acuity, Dr. X. did not feel excessive stress—the department was busy but not atypical.

  As mentioned in the text, giving environmental context affirms the potential impact this has on every ED patient.

- Important findings were called to Dr. X. by Dr. Y. It is commendable to have a process to have direct communication between radiologists and providers with all abnormal, high-risk findings.

  Commend communication and a process that requires it! Further, review this to determine if the communication process could be improved (made more comprehensive or efficient [SBAR?])

- The total time between order and completion of the head CT was 3 hours. The Joint Commission Certified Stroke Center expectation from potential stroke patient CT order to reporting a radiological interpretation is 45 minutes. If the hospital ED radiology process is compared to this benchmark, then it was not achieved for this patient.

  Referring to an EB literature or specialty-specific guideline provides some objective framework to the review process; in this case, reference was to standard CVA criteria well known to EM.

- [excerpt from conversation with] Dr. Z. (neurosurgery) got the call ... from Dr. X. who informed him of the CT findings of a large subdural. He lives close and the patient got to the OR quickly. His other recollections are that the RN informed him that the patient was talking and that the primary RN was not seen when he entered the room, but another RN was there. Also, he recalls that no blood work had been done when he arrived. They had to give universal blood as there was no type and cross done. He also notes that the coagulation results were not available until well after the patient left the ER.
- Dr. X. reports excellent interaction with Dr. Z.
- Further comments from Dr. X.:
  - On the patient's presentation she agreed with the ESI level and noted that the patient presented with multiple, unrelated complaints and did not appear is extreme distress, but had findings that appeared consistent with her chronically ill status.
  - Dr. X. was called to the bedside when the patient returned from the CT scan and was decompensating; she reports that she did not know the result of the imaging at the time of intervention (intubation)—RSI medication was appropriate for ICH management.
  - Dr. X. also reports that the lab process was compromised. Labs including coagulation studies were redrawn and as noted in the timeline above the first INR report was after the CT dictation.
  - Two areas of improvement Dr. X. promoted would be (1) more attention to staffing activity and (2) the attention to monitoring the imaging and laboratory process, though she indicates that this is not usually an issue at the hospital.
- Commentary on the above discussion with Dr. X. This author would advocate that the attention or vigilance to tracking ancillary work completion should not ideally be a high focus of physician work but at times is necessary. At this hospital, the ED physician often performs extensive point of care and departmental quality control of all ED processes. It could be concluded that the chronic deviation from priority activities often compromises the main physician function of medical decision making and directing medical management and ultimately the departmental patient flow.

Summary of Successes:

Give credit when and where due. Affirmation of good events supports the fairness of the process as well as promotes an openness to subsequent peer reviews. It also reinforces positive processes within the ED.

1. Dr. X. should be commended for her efforts.
2. Dr. X. aggressively intervened with the patient's decompensation, was technically successful with intubation, and made timely and appropriate consultation.

Summary of Improvements:

1. None from physician management focus.
2. Compliance with medication reconciliation requires ongoing monitoring. It cannot be overemphasized that the errant documentation could be propagated throughout the hospitalization.
3. Serum blood glucose activity on this patient requires review.
4. Ongoing evaluation of activity between departments, ED and radiology, is required to maximize patient care outcomes.

System issues are often enmeshed within peer review—many process improvement /reliability activities evolve from reviewing single events.

PATIENT Z

Peer Review

This is a 6-year-old female with severe cerebral palsy and status post ventricular-abdominal shunt placement who presented to the ED with CC of decreased LOC/change in mental status. The patient was initially evaluated in a critical care room; evaluation included IV access, blood work; head CT and shunt series. The patient was transferred to an unmonitored room; head CT identified shunt obstruction anatomy; ED MD contacted Dr. X.; Dr. X. found the patient with signs of herniation in ED; the patient was taken to OR for shunt revision. Postoperatively the patient was found to have diminished from baseline brain activity and had a prolonged hospitalization.

In reviewing this case, I reviewed the ED chart as well as first days of inpatient care; I reviewed MD dictations; and I spoke with the ED MD and Dr. X. about the case.

This is the peer reviewer balance with understanding the physician situation and the aggressive patient advocate. The summary is divided into chart components and includes a review of the MDM (judgment). Note that the peer review does not rely only on the chart documentation, but approached the physician as well for confirmation of the care.

My findings:

1. ED MD medical record documentation: inadequate. There is minimal history documented on chart. This is a complex technology-dependent child—PMHx was noted only as "hx of CP with multiple shunt revisions." The triage RN noted more facts of PMHx than the ED MD. There is no documentation of the child's baseline activity/functioning as to compare the ED presentation with background. All information could have been obtained from family at bedside or via the EMR of prior multiple admissions.

Value in referring to the EMR from prior visits. Despite many drawbacks and even more naysayers, today's EMRs often allow for rapid access to past records—allowing for a more rapid understanding of the patient. A good rule is to use material in the review that the MD had access to during the time of care and event.

There is minimal documentation of physical examination. The child was initially placed in a critical care room for evaluation. Documentation of PE on Chart: "NAD" box is checked. A majority of PE are noted as "normal" in this CP patient. HEENT examination noted as "nml," the patient has dysconjugate gaze and nystagmus at baseline. Abdominal examination is noted as "normal," with no mention of GT site or multiple abdominal scars/surgeries. Extremities examination: Chart note is uninterpretable; the patient has baseline spasticity and contracture to extremities. There is no neurological examination documented by the MD on this child that was found to have CNS compromise.

There is no documentation of hospital course and no documentation of reevaluation of mental status or neurological activity. RN flow sheet does note reassessment of the patient multiple times during ED stay.

2. ED MD evaluation (use of testing/examinations): inadequate. The evaluation is completed with minimal specificity for the patient. There is no evidence of consideration of differential diagnosis for altered mental status which would include hydrocephalus, seizure activity, CNS infection/shunt infection, drug OD (antiepileptics) in this specific patient. Workup in ED includes standard blood work. No drug levels were ordered. In patients with VAS and fever, obtaining CSF should be considered for "r/o" infection and antibiotics should also be considered. There is no note that the MD considered this option.

Important to provide a thorough review of the charting as well as place this in a timeline c/w the care process such that the case flows for the other physician reviewers/group process.

3. ED MD judgment: inadequate. The ED MD completes the evaluation with minimal specificity for this child. At minimal expectation, the patient was evaluated, clinically judged to be stable; appropriate evaluation for shunt malfunction was ordered and completed; the MD notified the specialist on receiving the CT results and neurosurgery evaluated the patient within 3 hours of ED stay.

The ED MD underappreciated the severity of the child's illness. The MD notes the child to be in "NAD" and allowed the child to move from a critical care room to an unmonitored room. In conversation with Dr. X., ED MD minimized the status of the patient while reporting the CT results. On arriving at bedside, Dr. X. found the child posturing and comatose. There is no evidence that the patient was reevaluated by the ED MD after the initial evaluation (2+ hours) until prior to Dr. X's arrival (and the ED MD cannot confirm this). Dr. X. also stated that the family was told the monitor was turned off due to the low HR alarm continuing to sound. Unfortunately with herniation, the heart pattern becomes bradycardic.

Issue identified with staff. An aware and educated staff could mediate this issue but potentially compounded it with a lack of specific knowledge about the pathologic potential of the patient. The ED MD needs to lead the staff in promoting and communicating an awareness of concerns per patient during point of care.

Conclusion:

In conversation with Dr. X., it is clear her impression was that the child could have been herniating since symptoms began 3 days prior to ED arrival. Full decompensation occurred within the ED. Whether the outcome would be changed is uncertain, but it is the larger mission of the ED to emergently intervene with critically ill children, limiting morbidity and preventing mortality.

I am concerned about the clinical judgment of the ED MD in this case. As the chart was completed, I can only interpret as the ED MD underrecognized/ underappreciated the severity of illness with this patient. Technology-dependent, developmentally delayed children are extremely challenging patients to assess and manage. A high level of clinical skill is required and evidence of this ability is lacking with this case. It is also concerning that despite knowing the outcome of the patient, that being the child was taken emergently to the OR for shunt revision, the ED MD did not review his notes and provide additional dictation/addendum to the chart to clarify the process of the case. Failure to recognize the untoward event and/or clarify actions could be a result of cavalier behavior or lack of clinical knowledge. The former is unacceptable and the latter need to be addressed in the future.

Anthony Ferroggiaro, MD
EDQA representative

It is important to just be solid in criticism and call out the errors; the effort further strengthens the peer review and improvement culture. This does not inhibit the effort of clinical improvement; the physician after group review was encouraged/tracked for pediatric critical care review.

■ EXAMPLE OF RESPONSE LETTER FROM COLLEAGUE REFERRAL

As noted in the discussion on peer review, closing the loop on either a referral or a triggered chart review is essential though time consuming. Writing a letter responding to complaints about patient care is important for several reasons as embedded within the letter: an indication that the group wants to improve and has a process for this; taking a colleague's concerns seriously; clearly a business sense of encouraging patient channels; and finally trying to evoke a culture of continuous performance improvement and patience. Sometimes you get to defend your colleagues! Not included within this letter but would further strengthen the conclusion is reference to articles supporting the care. Form letters are unacceptable in this profession; form to letters is good writing.

Dr. A.:

Thank you for referring the patient case. As QA representative for the Emergency Department, I have reviewed the case and discussed the case with my colleague, Dr. X.

Ms. T, a patient of your colleague, Dr. B., presented to the ED with complaints of shortness of breath and left arm pain. Over the past day, the patient had suffered from severe chest pain as well.

Dr. X's evaluation included a history that the patient had gone to water aerobics that day and then still feeling poorly presented to the ED. Extracted from the chart record, Dr. X. noted the patient was without chest pain in the ED, but had continued left arm pain. The past medical history documented is congestive heart failure, diverticulitis, hypertension, anemia with history of transfusion, and recent gastrointestinal evaluations.

On examination, Dr. X. noted no evidence of CHF. Vital signs were within normal limits, with the exception of an increased RR and oxygen saturation of 94%.

Significant studies included CBC, chemistry, cardiac markers, coagulation studies, CXR, and ECG. Therapy included ASA and a nitroglycerin infusion titrated to provide pain relief. The patient was admitted to telemetry for a "rule-out MI." The first cardiac indices were normal.

From your letter you expressed concern with Dr. X's history. You relate that he "misrepresented" the patient to your during the phone conversation. Moreover, you state that the patient's physical examination was not consistent with Dr. X's examination, that being the question of whether the patient was in congestive heart failure or not. I will try to address both these issues.

First, it is unclear whether the patient had a good understanding of her disease processes. On the ED coversheet, the triage RN only noted HTN and CHF as PMH. Under medications, the RN noted "water pill" and "blood pressure pill." Often, as you know, physicians are given limited information by the patients and must make best use of what is given. This is especially true in emergency medicine in which time is often limited. It is obvious that Dr. X. had to review the patient's record to obtain the information for his noted chart PMH. Also noted was a request for medical records. Often the old records do not arrive prior to the patient's admission to the hospital.

Due to the above problems, often the ED MD may have to decide disposition prior to complete knowledge of the patient and speak with a PCP (or the on-call MD). There is conflict when the on-call MD does not know the patient.

This is an ongoing issue with emergency medicine—the physician on-call for the group has no relationship with some of the patients and also cannot access the group's records to assist the ED MD.

It is also the responsibility of the internal medicine physicians to clarify the history and to "fine-tune" the medical care during the following hours and days of hospitalization.

In summary, though Dr. X. may not have had all the PMH on the patient at the time of communicating with you, the patient still received maximal, appropriate care.

Secondly, you have questioned Dr. X's physical examination. Per the record, Dr. X. noted no evidence of congestive heart failure in the chart. He even noted such in his discussion and disposition. From your letter, you were informed that night that the patient had evident CHF. Yet, in reviewing the complete medical record, including the admitting H&P, the hospitalist does not document CHF on examination, nor does she discuss it in her assessment and plan. Moreover, in the first 24 hours of hospitalization, no therapy for CHF is given. In fact, not much change in management is provided different from what is initiated in the ED. No diuresis is provided and the "ins and outs" for the first day indicate a positive intake. Moreover, your partner, Dr. B., in his morning note states "no sx of CHF."

In summary, the patient was not in congestive heart failure on admission from the ED. Dr. X. did not "misrepresent" the patient's physical examination....

To conclude, there are obvious differences in the care and communication of this patient.

Medicine is a challenging art. Often there is huge difficulty in getting adequate timely history while deciding direction of care. As I stated above, this is especially true for emergency medicine. On a personal note, in my 2 years working at X Hospital and 1 year of reviewing cases for my departments QA, I have been impressed at how well we, emergency physicians, do with what little information we are given in the short time we "know" the patient. We immensely benefit from PCP input, including a pre-patient presentation phone call, as well as the feedback you have given in the letter.

I will forward my findings to Dr. X. As far as background, Dr. X. has completed [xxxxxxx] emergency medicine residency. He is well trained […].

Sincerely,
Anthony A Ferroggiaro, MD
Emergency Department QA

■ SUMMARY OF ACTION ITEMS FOR PROCESS IMPROVEMENT FROM A RETROSPECTIVE CHART REVIEW

Action Plan	Target Date	Responsible Party—Title
Inventory radios and reevaluated the effectiveness of using walkie-talkies to contact ED nursing assistants.	XXXXX	
Acquire 10 new phones and develop exchange schedule to ensure half of phones are being charged while other half in use.	XXXXX	
	(Continued)	

Action Plan	Target Date	Responsible Party—Title
Develop structured communication guidelines (script) for the use of radios and wireless phones in the emergency room for communication between unit clerk, nursing techs, RNs, and physicians. SOP to require 1:1 focus of communication and acknowledgment of receipt. No zone pages.	XXXXX	
Standardize the communication between CT technician and ED nurses so that consistent staff member is responsible for initiating patient transfer for stat CT regardless of shift.	XXXXX	
Night manager attending radiology staff meetings working toward enhancement of and handoff communication between CT tech and ED RN each time the patient is transferred to and from radiology.		
Work with individual staff nurse on time management, importance of notifying charge nurse when he or she needs help, using the tracking board regularly to monitor pending tests and completion verification, and following RN-RN structured handoff communication process.	XXXXX	
Promote and sustain the same culture among all ED nurses.		
Review the blood-draw escalation process for reliable follow-up when unable to obtain a sample. Determine a way to improve transparency when collection step is completed the way lab-order time and lab-process time are automatically tracked.	XXXXX	

■ TRANSITION—THE EFFECTIVENESS OF PEER REVIEW

Is peer review successful? This depends on the organization's goals. The goals may be compliance with a minimal program to achieve TJC requirements or to have some program to replace those physician "bad apples" or a method embedded within a larger quality improvement program that heightens practice through interesting or triggered cases and applauding or demanding higher quality of practice.

Jamtvedt et al.[15] conclude that audit and feedback (defined as a summary of clinical performance over time) could be effective in improving professional practice. This was affirmed in another Cochrane Review[16] by similar authors. More specifically, the authors found that feedback "may be more effective when baseline performance is low, the source is a supervisor or colleague, it is provided more than once, it is delivered in both verbal and written formats, and when it includes both explicit targets and an action plan" (Table 2-5). Many of these elements are described above and within Chapter 3, Sequential Clinical Auditing.

■ **TABLE 2-5.** Peer Review Feedback—Increasing the Success

Increasing Success With Practice Change Through Peer Review Feedback

1. Low baseline performance
2. Source of feedback is colleague or supervisor
3. Increased frequency of feedback
4. Verbal and written feedback
5. Action plan and agreed upon targets

Used with permission. Ivers N, J. G. (2012). Audit and feedback: Effects on Professional Practice and Healthcare Outcomes. Cochrane Database of Systematic Reviews(6). doi:10.1002/14651858.
Note: Most elements present in the SCA structure.

A fundamental problem with the current peer review method known to many organizations and groups is that the volume of cases reviewed is an inadequate learning method and an inadequate representation a physician's complete practice. Like all review systems, current peer review is dependent on the mechanism of entering cases into review; in the case of emergency medicine, most systems have entry points for chart review from simple referrals by other physicians to set triggers such as return visits within 72 hours and/or all mortalities associated with the emergency department. In 2007, I reviewed the frequency of peer review cases per physician within our 75-physician group and determined that on average less than 1% of the physician's practice was represented through peer review. I suspect this is the community pattern due to (1) our use of standard review triggers, (2) Edwards' survey that peer chart review is the most common form of review method, and (3) other sources note a similar frequency.[6]

Even more impressive, the range of cases reviewed per physician resulted in several physicians receiving zero chart reviews during 1 or more years (Figures 2-15 and 2-16). Thus, dependent on the established triggers for peer review, some

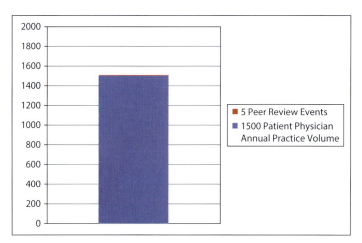

FIGURE 2-16. Representation (to scale) of average annual peer review cases to physician practice volume.

physicians would have no individual clinical performance evaluation throughout 1 year if the group relied solely on the standard retrospective chart review triggers. Obviously, with the inherent goal of continuous improvement, all physicians would expect some review of practice that is objective and beyond their own day to day self-review. Again, probably the reason for the narrow triggers (small nets) is the decision to limit work review, concern for time and cost of nonclinical activity, and a business decision to achieve compliance but not quality improvement. There is a need to get to a method that is more representative of the complete physician practice, a structured, larger sample that can represent a comprehensive view of the physician's work.

Moreover, peer review is individual, or case specific. Reviewing a case in isolation is problematic as it may result in bias due to an unnecessary, excessive emphasis on a single outcome. The reviewed physician may respond in several ways; there may be a tendency to overrespond with future cases, perhaps moving toward overtesting or overtreating (defensive) and the result is a practice movement outside of evidence-based practice. The isolated case and excessive emphasis has the potential to result in the reviewed physician developing a heightened emotionally negative response in general to his/her career causing the proverbial "more harm than good." Another complication would be within the group, the potential to view the involved physician's practice as generally compromised when few cases out of 2000 annual cases are hardly representative of the quality of the clinical work. This is nicely paralleled in Berenson's critique of CMS' PQRS system but pertains here.[17] Conversely a balanced, holistic, sequential review can avoid this unnecessary, isolated judgment and deflation. Any clinical review should be affirmative that the physician is practicing in a challenging environment in which success is not expected to be 100% but that the goal is continual learning and continual improvement and one or a few cases do not define a physician's practice quality.

A group should not *only* perform retrospective chart review but should have a strong program of clinical quality improvement.[1,14] There are two additional reasons beyond the betterment of care and the calibration of provider or group practice as discussed above that should be mentioned. First, mere compliance with retrospective chart review and no other quality improvement program does not achieve differentiation between the current group and other groups (including CMGs) that

---

■ **TABLE 2-6.** Value of Comprehensive Clinical Review (Sequential Clinical Auditing)

Value of Comprehensive Clinical Review (Sequential Clinical Auditing)

1. More effective individual care improvement method
2. Group care improvement method
3. Knowledge translation method
4. Group to group differentiation in the market (brand)
5. Internal marketing of group practice quality for contract stability
6. Potential market growth due to branding (high quality with proof)

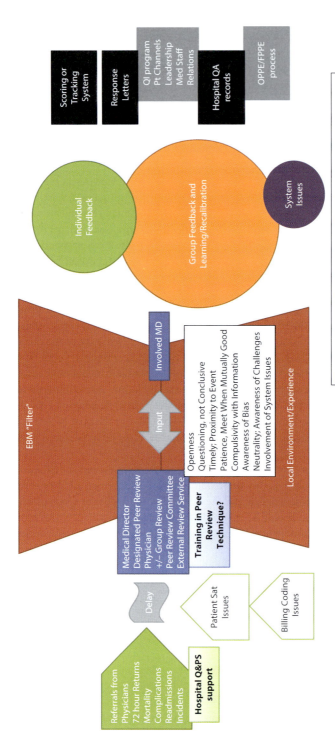

FIGURE 2-17. Summary of the peer review process.

may want the health system emergency medicine contract. Similarly, most institutions are achieving high, near equivalent scores with CMS core measures such that this program is hardly differentiating. In competitive medical care, departments or groups need to ensure contract stability and longevity. A program in quality improvement can be a strategic strong point during contract negotiations especially if it aligns with established or developing service lines. Second, associated with advertising your value and contract stability, routine retrospective chart review (as most facilities achieve it[1] results in administration or medical staff leaders (CMO, CEO) receiving only negatively toned data and leading to potential misinterpretation of the practice group's quality. Wise executives can look past the individual and/or sum of the cases and realize the process is skewed to look for errors. Others may develop a negative outlook on the clinical quality of the practice, which when combined with the chronically poor patient satisfaction scores associated with emergency services (in unequal comparison to other outpatient services) potentially could trigger a demand for action and/or replacement. Wise group or department leadership introduces group successes at upper level meetings and with health system leadership. In short, find (create) and promote your strengths. Aggressive differentiation is redefining the playing field, publicizing a novel comprehensive, self-derived, specialty-driven metrics and taking the lead on value as well as taking the lead in the hospital or health system and the region. A strong clinical quality improvement program (sequential clinical auditing) can supply the data and the positive points for this conversation/marketing (Table 2-6).

A Summary of the peer review process is included in Figure 2-17.

REFERENCES

1. Edwards MT, Benjamin EM. The process of peer review in US hospitals. *JCOM*. 2009;461-467.

2. The Joint Commission. *Electronic standards manual*. (March 6, 2012). Retrieved on December 17, 2013, from http://e-dition.jcrinc.com.

3. Chan LS, Elabiad M, Zheng L, et al. A medical staff peer review system in a public teaching hospital–an internal quality improvement tool. *J Healthc Qual*. 2012;36(1):37-44.

4. The Joint Commission. *JC Physician Blog*. August 21, 2013. http://www.jointcommission.org/jc_physician_blog/oppe_fppe_tools_privileging_decisions/.

5. Dellinger RP. Surviving Sepsis Campaign guidelines for management of severe sepsis and septic shock. *Crit Care Med*. 2004;32(3):858-873.

6. Lovett PB, Massone, RJ. Rapid response team activations within 24 hours of admission from the emergency department: an innovative approach for performance improvement. *Acad Emerg Med*. 2014;21(6):667-672.

7. Croskerry P. The feedback sanction. *Acad Emerg Med*. 2000;7(11):1232-1238.

8. Berstein SL. The effect of emergency department crowding on clinically oriented outcomes. *Acad Emerg Med*. 2009;16(1):1-10.

9. Hoot N. Systematic review of emergency department crowding: causes, effects, and solutions. *Ann Emerg Med*. 2008;52(2):126-136.

10. Orlander JD, Barber TW, Fincke BG. The morbidity and mortality conference: the delicate nature of learning from error. *Acad Med.* 2002;77(10):1001-1006.

11. Orlander JD, Fincke BG. Morbidity and mortality conference: a survey of academic internal medicine departments. *J Gen Int Med.* 2003;18(8):656-658.

12. Peterson P. Teaching peer review. *JAMA.* 1973;224(6):884-885.

13. Rosen H. Making peer review more productive. *JAMA.* 1983;224(6):2305-2306.

14. Sanazaro P. Medical audit, continuing medical education and quality assurance. *West J Med.* 1976;125(3):241-252.

15. Jamtvedt G, Young JM, Kristoffersen DT, O'Brien MA, Oxman AD. Does telling people what they have been doing change what they do? A systematic review of the effects of audit and feedback. *Qual Saf Health Care.* 2006;15(6):433-436.

16. Ivers N, Jamtvedt G, Flottorp S, et al. Audit and feedback: effects on professional practice and healthcare outcomes. *Cochrane Database Syst Rev.* 2012;(6):1-4. doi:10.1002/14651858.

17. Berenson RA. Grading a physician's value–the misapplication of performance measurement. *N Engl J Med.* 2013;369(22):2079-2081.

Sequential Clinical Auditing

■ INTRODUCTION

The clinical audit is not a new tool in the evaluation of physician performance.[1] The definition, obtained from the National Institute for Health and Care Excellence glossary,[2] is a process for monitoring standards of clinical care to see if it is being carried out in the best way possible. The result of such a generalized description is a wide interpretation and titling of activity representing clinical auditing including standard peer review. Others often relate auditing to medical risk management activities.

For this text, clinical auditing is a method of reviewing the clinical activity around the decision making or actions related to disease presentations and/or procedures and comparing group and individual work to established standards. In short, it is disease- or chief complaint-specific comprehensive practice review, linked or grounded in evidence-based medicine.

As in the following examples, clinical auditing is an organized method of clinical review based on a predetermined focus. The auditors select a disease entity requiring review, select the parameters to identify a number of cases, review these according to a predetermined standard (either established by the group or obtained from external sources), and provide feedback on practice accuracy (with standards) to all physicians associated with the cases (Figures 3-1 and 3-2).

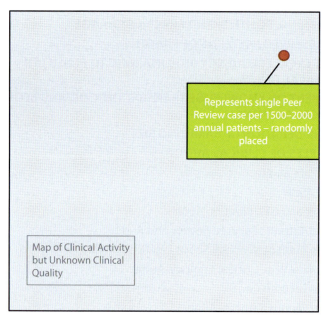

Represents single Peer Review case per 1500–2000 annual patients – randomly placed

Map of Clinical Activity but Unknown Clinical Quality

FIGURE 3-1. Model representation of peer review case to overall clinical practice (not to scale).

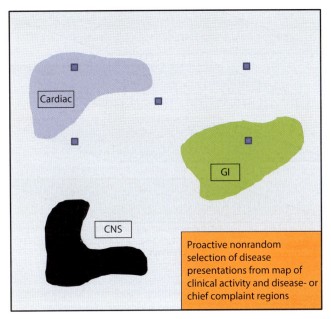

FIGURE 3-2. Model representation of sequential clinical auditing to overall clinical practice (not to scale).

When combined as a sequence of audits of specific complaints or disease processes in a comprehensive program, audits provide a more holistic, accurate view of a physician's and a group's clinical performance. The author, being such a woefully creative person, will title this type of "linked-audit" structure as sequential clinical auditing (SCA). In the framework of quality improvement, SCA is a comprehensive feedback mechanism on practice performance that any organization or department can achieve. If framed as research, these are similar to observational studies on clinical practice according to disease presentation.

As described in Chapter 2, standard peer review is usually initiated due to a complaint or a questionable outcome. Based on the process, peer review is largely an emotionally negative, reactionary endeavor in quality assurance. Rarely are groups promoting interesting cases to be reviewed in this method of peer review and as triggers for knowledge gain (translation). Sequential clinical auditing avoids this problem through the proactive selection of disease presentations or procedures; thus, the opportunity for clinical improvement often arises in a positive background and not from an "error." This method becomes even stronger with an organized schedule of audits; the first quarter is a planned focus on chest pain, the second quarter is abdominal pain, and the third could be airway interventions. A published, agreed upon schedule allows for openness to the process.

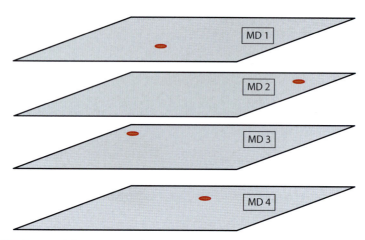

FIGURE 3-3. Model representing four physicians and randomness of peer case review over time—single cases in isolation and minimal if any group benefit.

A structured approach to clinical auditing also allows for a positive view within the group. No longer does the physician feel like every case may be "targeted" for the peer review "trial" and then tends toward practicing in a defensive mode. Instead, all physicians are evaluated simultaneously and equally (Figures 3-3 and 3-4). With the development of a comprehensive program as a series of audits, the physician actually knows what is currently being audited and what will in the future. This level of practice improvement transparency allows for the physicians to support the auditing efforts and allows for an openness to consider practice change. I have observed that it also behaviorally affects physicians, unconsciously or consciously the awareness of the topics or foci of the sequential clinical audit modifies care even prior to data and discussion (a Hawthorne effect). It also allows for the group rather than one individual organizer to direct the focus of clinical improvement.

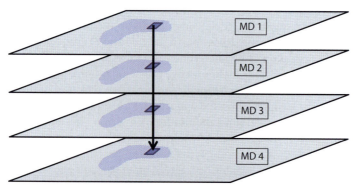

FIGURE 3-4. Model of SCA—simultaneous clinical auditing of cardiac presentation in all physicians (example includes four physicians).

Inclusively, the trigger for clinical auditing of a specific population of patients can be initiated from a singular peer review but the collection of the cases will be of a larger scope. An example, one physician has a difficult pyelonephritis case and the clinical auditing trigger would be pyelonephritis or UTI or DM/pyelonephritis or urosepsis and sepsis response. This may even be from the established peer review triggers but instead of assessing one case, that case becomes one in a collection of cases about a disease process (Figure 3-5). The resulting audit may determine several physicians in the group have similar gaps in knowledge or method (as expected) and thus many benefit from the one event.

This point cannot be overstated (but I will try). Considering each physician is fallible and has gaps in knowledge and low points in technique or practice quality, an appropriate assumption is that what challenges one physician will often challenge several. SCA provides an opportunity for group practice review that peer review cannot achieve. These two methods have totally different penetrations on practice change. The concept manifest in the SCA process is that all physicians should be assessed simultaneously and equally resulting in individual impact, group awareness and learning, and potentially group oversight and behavioral pressure to change (Figure 3-4).

Finally in many of the groups that I was associated with, there was no formal group learning approach. The peer-reviewed physician oftentimes only discussed the case with the medical director in a one-on-one private manner. Understandably,

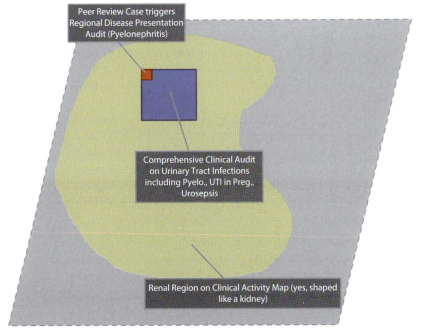

FIGURE 3-5. Relationship to peer chart review as a trigger for clinical auditing.

if the effort was to protect the physician's ego rather than the next patient who presents similarly to the department—this was a good system! But hypothesizing that many physicians have similar gaps in knowledge and care approaches and that the "mistake" could potentially be repeated due to the limited collective learning for the group, then the ultimate goal of patient safety and increasing practice value and outcomes might not be met with an isolated approach. The likelihood based on the nature of emergency medicine that the patient will present with a similar problem but to a different physician is high and without collective knowledge or learning then the result of a less than ideal response is greater. Publishing the clinical audits combined with group presentations allows for information transfer and the discussion leads to a heightened practice awareness within the group.

Clinical auditing is a stronger clinical improvement form based on:

- The subject matter or foci of clinical audits are disease states or processes of clinical practice, not individual case peer review (Table 3-1).
- This is a proactive method of quality improvement since it does not rely on untoward events to trigger reviews. Though it is not a random sampling of a population, due to the volume of cases and sampling method it is more representative of a physician's practice. See Sampling Addendum.
- The group or practice has clinically managed the patients, thus the data and the outcomes in the comparison are owned by the group and by the individuals. This has a big impact (see Publishing, Politics, and Practice Change section) on the openness to consider changing practice as well as the interest in participating in the process of auditing with recommendations and other support.
- Mechanistically SCA is the effort to connect the actions within a local medical practice environment to the standards promoted in evidence-based medicine. Individually, physicians often consider their practices as standard of care without much evidence to support *or* challenge this assumption. SCA can provide a direct comparison of the local practice standard to the literature-based advisement of care.
- Working at a group level increases acceptance compared to the tendency of individuals to be defensive with the review of single peer cases. As suggested previously, peer review has inherent weaknesses as a method of performance

■ TABLE 3-1. A Comparison of Clinical Auditing and Peer Chart Review

Clinical Auditing	Peer Review Method
Identify a disease/procedure focus.	Identify single case.
Review many patient opportunities.	Review one patient opportunity.
Review many MDs involved.	Review one physician.
Data organized for individual and group feedback.	Knowledge distribution potential but limited.
Events can be sequential and cyclical.	Events are only singular.

improvement; the opportunity to look collectively (with or without anonymity) at a disease presentation at the group level reduces defensiveness.

- The data are granular enough to be reflective of individual practice when combined with sequence or series of audits involving several clinical presentations or foci. This achieves larger value to the individual who can look at a series of cases and realize either satisfactory care or opportunity for improvement rather than rely on the singular case in peer review to be reflective of practice pattern. An example of this is reviewing the intubation success of each physician in the group over 1 year compared to one peer review event involving a challenging intubation. Physicians are trained to consider trends as more valuable data than single events.

■ WHAT SEQUENTIAL CLINICAL AUDITING IS NOT

SCA is not patient satisfaction or CMS core measure work. As stated in the introduction, physicians often complain about the imbalanced hospital or health system administrative focus on patient satisfaction. Both groups are correct to advocate for *medical treatment and hospitality* as mutual goals for patients. The irony though is that few physician groups work to provide a strong system of clinical performance or outcome data that could provide a more complete picture of health care (on the medical treatment side) and thereby balance the administrative focus on patient satisfaction and hospitality (Figure 3-6).

CMS Core Measurement tracking and reporting is commonplace due to the compliance requirements for CMS reimbursement. Understandably, since the issue is reimbursement and a focus of the participants on health care, and since CMS is the "majority insurer" nationwide, the physicians and groups are obliged to attend to these issues. Unfortunately, like the current peer review practiced in many groups, it is unlikely that the number of clinical cases involving the Core Measures will represent a comprehensive picture of the physician's annual work.[3,4] Thus CMs cannot be the only method of clinical review of practice and groups should avoid this narrow approach and superficial review.

Most of these CMs are largely operational measures and have less focus on clinical practice decisions or physician activity. Indeed, many health systems in

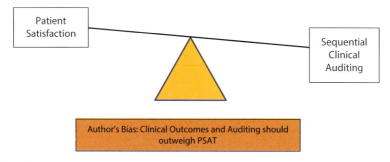

FIGURE 3-6. Balancing patient satisfaction with clinical auditing.

order to achieve compliance (the base form of quality) have removed physician decision making in many of the CMs (automatic blood cultures in pneumonia patients and protocols for ECGs on literally everyone). A comprehensive clinical audit program with operational extension has the ability to regain the physician practice authority that is necessary for operational efficiency within the department (see below in The Operational Impact of Auditing).

Moreover, as described in Chapter 2, the likelihood that anything legislated or externally demanded/driven will amount to more than compliance is low.[5,6] More astounding is the opposite effect that is observed in some emergency departments. The gross effort to achieve compliance results in increased cost, wasted time, and wasted activity. One example of many is the effort to achieve ECGs on the TJC measure to achieve the 90-minute PCI window on STEMIs as well as the CMS' PQRS program of obtaining ECGs on all nontrauma CP presentations age >40 has resulted in policies of obtaining ECGs on *all* patients presenting with chest pain.

Still, there is hope. Measures do not have to be approached in isolation. Another value to the SCA method is the ease of embedding the CMS CM elements (similar to the use of peer review cases to trigger a focus [Figure 3-5]) within an audit or audit series. Consider an audit on NSTEMI management which is not associated with the STEMI CM. Since these patients are often clinically underappreciated on entry to the clinical arena,[7] clearly benefit from early recognition and specific care pathways and many of these patients may present with chest pain mimics, the audit could review the timeliness of ECG in this group as well as the frequency of medication administration (Figure 3-7). This effort can achieve simultaneous, mutual goals.

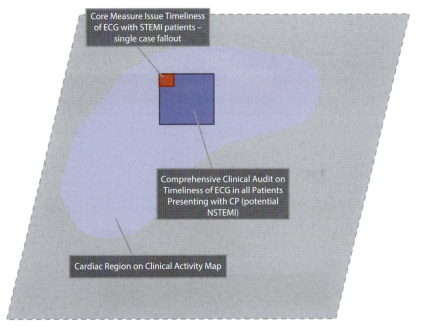

Core Measure Issue Timeliness of ECG with STEMI patients – single case fallout

Comprehensive Clinical Audit on Timeliness of ECG in all Patients Presenting with CP (potential NSTEMI)

Cardiac Region on Clinical Activity Map

FIGURE 3-7. Relationship of core measure focus with clinical auditing.

Many reviewing the SCA method would summarize that this is another physicians' report card or similar to profiling. In truth any auditing process is dependent on the group or business philosophy, structure, and objectives. Any group can profile its participants/employees/partners and have outcomes of this profiling as a spectrum of nonpunitive openness and improvement to a lack of promotion, income compromise or at worst cause for job insecurity. Beyond the goal differences, there are process differences with SCA from other report cards. SCA, as proposed, is a method that is driven *within* the physician group and assisted perhaps through single or several physicians such as a medical director. Every physician has gaps in knowledge and technical skills—the audit process allows the group to assist the individual in continuous clinical improvement for the betterment of the group. Those who administer the audit process must be careful to not present as policing or distinguishing themselves as better. This will be further discussed in "Publishing, politics, and practice change" and in Chapter 5. Moreover, SCA is not an external requirement compared with CM compliance or other hospital-based medical staff efforts.[6] External demands do not allow for internal discussion and transparency. SCA emphasizes autonomy of a group in deciding the review foci as well as employing the group to determine the expectations of local care based on literature review and audit data comparison.

Balanced scorecards are rarely balanced. In contrast to the strength of SCA due to its comprehensiveness, most balanced scorecards have minimal technical data on each physician as the sources are CM and peer review and thus are criticized as nonrepresentative. Scorecards or report cards often are not structured to provide feedback for improvement as they include macrometrics like general CT usage and are not granular or specific. In addition, the data are poorly represented in absolute and not within the methods and background of statistical process control.

Taken from the patient's perspective, the patient generically considers the emergency department as part of the hospital or even the community. Infrequently, the patient comes to a particular emergency department due to a specific physician with privileges or due to a prior interaction. An example of this would be a postoperative question for the patient's surgeon, the patient returns to the site of the surgery and not necessarily due to the EM physician present. Secondly, the shift pattern structure of EM physician work is usually inconsistent; thus the patient with prior ED experience expects to interact with whoever is working that shift. The result is that external profiling of individual EM physicians does not add value for the patient.

Finally, when the patient is in pain or in a life-threatening situation it is unlikely that he or she is not considering the prior interaction with an emergency physician as cause for bypassing a hospital. Indeed, the CMS Hospital Compare Website states, "In an emergency, you should go to the nearest hospital" on its screen.[8] The irony is that the program does not have geolocation and mapping directions—consider timeliness of care!

■ THE OPERATIONAL IMPACT OF AUDITING

Most departmental operational activities are efforts to manage more patients over time; the literature is full of patient-volume management articles and pragmatically the world is such that more patients are coming to the emergency

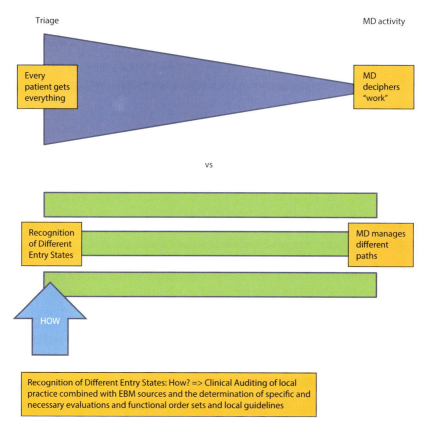

Triage

MD activity

Every patient gets everything

MD deciphers "work"

vs

Recognition of Different Entry States

MD manages different paths

HOW

Recognition of Different Entry States: How? => Clinical Auditing of local practice combined with EBM sources and the determination of specific and necessary evaluations and functional order sets and local guidelines

FIGURE 3-8. Effort to "press the machine" do all for everyone.

department for medical care.[9] Many departments consider efficiency as doing everything on every patient, just trying to do it faster.[10] An example is that every chest pain patient gets an ECG and a marker panel of troponin, BNP, D-dimer, etc (Figure 3-8). Unfortunately many departments are not considering that much of what is done may be valueless. Even point-of-care testing is not faster if testing in itself is not needed.[11,12] The main problem relates to the concept of opportunity cost; doing one action precludes simultaneously doing another. Not doing a valueless action often allows time to complete a different action of potentially more value. Operational efficiency is about sequencing a more valued series of actions.

Another way this activity can be economically described is using the *law of diminishing returns* (Figure 3-9). The physician or program that controls the value-added activity with each patient has the potential to stay early in the curve of the diagram, thereby potentially maximizing value (reimbursement, health, safety, etc) for LOS minute. If the patient has increasing LOS due to valueless activity, then the stay moves along the curve in time and diminishing gain per LOS minute occurs. This may not be operationally evident in POCT but is evident in the LOS

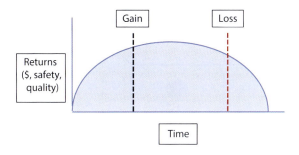

Consider:

Gain – No CT imaging for CHI who is age appropriate, no anticoagulation, normal mental status

Loss – Non-EBM decision to image, CT imaging queue, interpretation, transcription, recognition by EM MD

Conversely, think of the gain of creating another earlier open room and new patient evaluation.

FIGURE 3-9. Simplified law of diminishing returns.

between unnecessary CT imaging and those patients receiving no imaging[13] and the frequency of CT imaging in general.[10]

Contrast this with some departments having overwhelming time goals such as a fixed x-hour average LOS to maintain a position early in the curve. Unfortunately, the department too often only addresses a time goal and misses the opportunity to provide quality care. This system response was well described with the NHS 4-hour rule.[14] The result is that every shift a physician is told, "I was here yesterday" or "two days ago" and "I am not better." A balanced approach can occur but managers have to consider the whole system (Figure 3-10).

As above, in this effort to push the patient-processing machine faster, clinical accuracy and efficiency are ignored, presumed, or reduced to a secondary priority. It has become a game of numbers and not value. Yet the review of clinical activity with focus on accuracy and efficiency should be the basis for operational goals. There are several possible reasons for avoiding a focus on clinical efficiency and accuracy (Table 3-2).

First, this is (still) a pay-for-procedure world and supposedly the physician will get paid less for less activity; the resulting culture is to test more. The irony here is that sometimes auditing shows that more testing is required as in the Neonatal Sepsis Audit (see examples of audits) in which more LPs were advocated and more admissions of the 31- to 60-day-old neonates were a result of more evaluations aligned with EBM. Critics about pay-for-performance and critics about pay-for-procedure could realize this activity is about increasing value while replacing a less-valued action with a more or most valued action, but activity (and billing) is

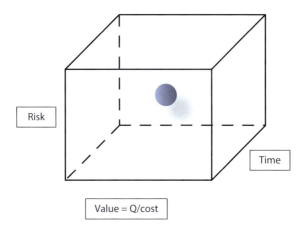

There is operational worth with envisioning goals within a multi-dimensional model as the distortion of one value is more obvious with the manipulation of another value in isolation. As in the example above, shortening the time length or LOS has the potential to raise the risk of missing a pathological process as well as impacting value. Similarly balancing risk may cause LOS to increase.

FIGURE 3-10. Balanced goal approach for increased value.

often conserved. The vision must also be extended into the patient continuum and beyond the focused point-of-care interaction; doing a more valued activity may mean earlier return to health or less return visits to the follow-up PCP, or even less medication interactions.

Second, patients mistakenly think (or are led to believe) that any action done adds value to their medical care and their "demand for medical care" promotes testing. The fallacy here is that the least scientifically and technically knowledgeable are determining activity. Systems that allow this "choice" are misinterpreting patient-centered care. The result is that the testing is varied and wide in the value spectrum without a process to clarify direction. Unfortunately acquiescing to a patient compromises the whole department if it is repetitively done. In some odd behavioral way, doing more testing, putting a patient at risk, results in the potential (or the assumption) for better patient satisfaction scores (remember patients cannot see the radiation [sarcasm]). Again, there is an imbalance toward patient satisfaction and a circular argument that drives this issue.

■ **TABLE 3-2.** Why Clinical Accuracy and Efficiency Is a Secondary Priority

1. The world is still pay-for-procedure.
2. Patients think doing something adds value.
3. A lack of physician-centric model in operational decision making.
4. EM physician inconsistent presence within the institution and lacking a "voice" in operations.
5. Health care business structure reduces physician clinical leadership.

The third reason is the lack of a physician-centric model of EM decision making (DM). Physician activity is the keystone to ED operational efficiency (good or bad) as the physician is the main authority of action in the department. Unfortunately most departments do not link operational activity directly to core physician activity but create layers of processes as workarounds to address the inconsistent EM physician presence and clinical advocacy. The reason for this is due to the current structural and political dynamic within the department and an aspect of the behavior or EM physicians as a specialty.

Regardless of the business and legal structure of the group, most EM physicians at a site are not involved in the management of a department's operational processes and clinical outcomes. The emergency medicine physician's inconsistent presence due to shift work and solo decision making while on shift automatically adds variation within a practice site.[15] The efforts to manage this variability usually result in weaker processes and more inefficiency. For example, nonspecific triage order sets for the presentation of chest pain when applied to every patient with chest pain results in dramatic inefficiencies; yet these order sets were developed (often through passive physician acceptance) to minimize the impact of physician variation (Monday it was physician X's approach but Tuesday it was physician Y's) and due to the volume-flow pressure in the department.

Amplifying this problem many medical directors and other administrative personnel approach operational problems by applying mimics and general remedies without fully understanding their clinical culture or system. An example of departments focusing on one, isolated metric for improvement is the placement of midlevel providers in triage in order to reduce the time-to-provider metric.[16,17] Unfortunately these providers also initiate care/orders that are often clinically less aligned with the literature than an emergency physician, resulting in overtesting and inappropriate testing, most obvious in the higher acuity patients.[16] In this case, the leadership's operational metric focus compromises departmental clinical accuracy and efficiency.

Finally, the current health care structure does not support the MD position, whereas if recognized there should be effort to reinforce based on patient value. In the goal of obtaining a wide experience base, I have worked for (subjected myself to) several national contract management groups (CMGs) as well as private practice groups. Part of the loss of physician-centric activity is due to weak contractual linkage. The independent contractor (IC) role that many CMGs and other practices promote results in EM physicians feeling less "ownership" of the department's outcomes and are less incentivized to promote EBM within the department (it is just 8, 9, 10 hours of shift work!). Conversely, there is a dynamic triangle of power and an increased contractual focus between the CMG and the health system or hospital resulting in a weakening of the physician "voice" at times (Figure 3-11). Ironically, these CMGs promote the independence, but it is that independence that weakens their business stability (contract flux, struggle to staff the department, disinterest by physicians) and operational efficiency. Due to the physician-patient relationship which directly impacts health value and is linked to revenue, these organizations should be reinforcing a physician-centric model! Unfortunately

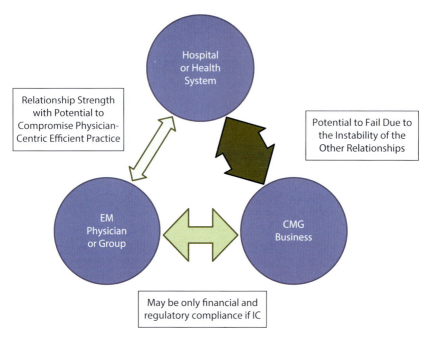

FIGURE 3-11. Common triangle dynamic in health care.

I have also witnessed the negatives of partnership and the lack of interest and responsiveness to change that "partners-for-life" express. No job should be protected "for life" when lives are at stake and with science driving innovation. Groups may struggle with technical stagnation as shown in the subsequent SCA example of the sepsis review. EM private practice often promotes autonomy to the detriment of flow, consistency and constancy of purpose of the whole departmental unit. The result of a shell of management, many private practice groups have weak strategic methods, largely being reactionary and often contract in presence when threatened rather than driving the relationship with administration with focus on clinical accuracy and proof of high-quality outcomes.

Alternatively but rarely, physicians have clarified an operational approach that embeds their collective decision making. One example is a more stratified chest pain workup at a local site; examples would be in the 20-year old with chest pain obtaining only an ECG or rhythm strip or chest pain in the elderly looking for Coumadin prescriptions and ordering the PT/INR (Figure 3-8). The physician group "sees" its local environment, compares it with published standards and through consensus or group process, advocates for a less variable, more specific (valued) practice. SCA is a tool that provides that vision.

High-quality, precise care starts *in the department meeting* in which the group decides, based on audits and reflection with EBM sources, how that disease presentation will be universally managed. This is not an acceptance of each physician's approach; rather the group's physicians collectively agree on care and thus can maintain consistency. This is different from most sites: allowing each physician to determine direction of care at the point of patient contact. The subsequent repeat clinical audit can reinforce that change and universal management.

The SCA foci are disease processes or medical complaints that structurally lead to activity review within the department and allow for direct reflection on the practice culture of the department. Indeed, SCA does not have to be an isolated loop feedback for physician technical activity. Instead the audit method provides an opportunity for the physician group to further define internally their individual practice but also to extend authority to the activities of other departmental personnel. The audits then could represent the physician "voice" in operations. Physicians (the group) should position themselves as the EBM resources and champions for their specialty and locality.*

Indeed, as per the following diagram, physician decision making has distinct impact zones throughout the ED evaluation and management process as well as affecting clinical practice beyond the borders of the ED, including pre- and post-ED management (Figure 3-12). Consider a traumatic neck pain/c-spine imaging audit. A modification of the physician practice toward use of the NEXUS criteria could impact the activity of the ED team; the RNs and MLs would learn to use the criteria in triage decision making or in order sets resulting in more specific (less variance) use of immobilization and imaging; the knowledgeable radiology tech and radiologist may provide oversight and risk management requiring a c-collar placement prior to completion of any imaging order; downstream physician practice could rely on the conserved process and move toward other issues in care. Overall efficiency again comes from a more value-laden sequence.

This concept goes beyond the implementation of clinical guidelines but describes a holistic or cultural process of practicing medicine within a department. The core is the change and collective physician advocacy of selective practice processes which may change over time due to continuous review, innovation, and change in local population disease patterns that emanates outward to impact all the participants of care. This ends up not being a paper menu list in triage for thoughtless practice.

In the future, health care performance might less be about core measures which are largely federal cost savings efforts and more about local differentiation. Clinical accuracy can be a method of competing for patients, insurers, contracts, and brand name. To be able to prove that one provides better care outcomes while being more efficient in the market has huge potential. We see bill boards for "faster" ERs but what are they basing "better" on and can they really prove they have better outcomes? Though emergency medicine is largely quiet on strategic market position, consider the opportunity or impact as a department (business unit) within the

---

*One critical observation is that having the medical director dictate an approach (EBM or not) is not the same as a group consensus. No individual's practice can fully represent the group. When the director is not clinically present on shift the other physicians practice differently to a muted benefit or cost. Just as each EM physician has varied technical ability, so do medical directors.

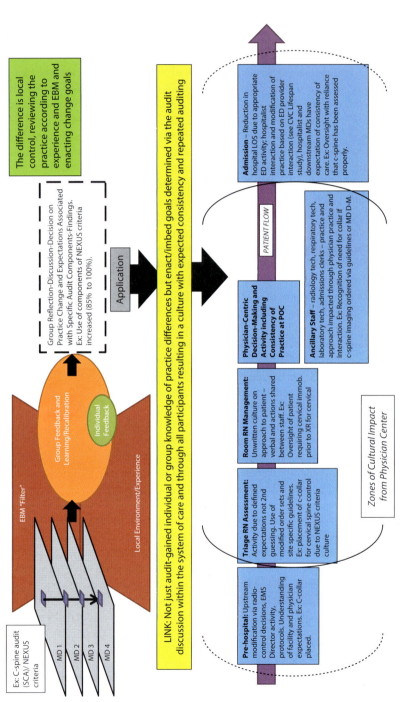

FIGURE 3-12. Relationship with SCA, EBM-aligned practice accuracy and operational impact through ED flow process.

health system and the potential role the emergency departments play within each organization, even simply the more efficient management of the 40% to 50% admissions that occur through the ED.

From an internal marketing standpoint, auditing provides an opportunity for the emergency department to technically lead within the facility. A strong clinical improvement program can be an aspect of dialogue during contract negotiations as well as between departments. A proactive approach to managing outcomes is a method that promotes job security for the group and the individual physicians.

■ MICHAEL PORTER AND SEQUENTIAL CLINICAL AUDITING: A STEP IN THE RIGHT DIRECTION

I am not sure what type or level of competition has a place in medical care. Personally I like to compete against infections, infarctions, hemorrhage, and the lack of oxygen.

Porter and Teisberg's[18] concept of "competition at the wrong level" distinctly relates to the three examples of hard quality described in this text. In today's health care there is an assumption of good care or value dependent on the name of the facility or group association (branding). In emergency medicine, competition is at the health system level as the service is hospital based. (Interesting to see what the stand-alone, nonaffiliated ED or UC will bring). Yet the focus of value, the patient condition, is not present within the structures of physician review. Peer chart review (PCR) is an example of Porter and Teisberg's "competition is too narrow" in which reviewing a discrete intervention with a single physician cannot be extrapolated with any certainty to the rest of the physician practice or to other patients presenting with the same medical condition. ABEM's APP PCPI requirement has potential if directed toward medical conditions or disease states but unfortunately the advocacy to date has been on operational processes that limit the activity to discrete actions.

SCA is a process that has the potential to step from the "level of discrete interventions" to the opportunity to view disease-process care and outcomes of the group. SCA directs the focus toward the medical condition and represents opportunity to act competitively at the right level of care (beyond the individual physician or action). Understandably it is necessary to decompose care or activity around the disease process, but as shown in the subaudits, recomposition of these actions to the physician and group level is obtainable. This activity is based on the need for accountability in the disease- or condition-management process but does not disallow or cause loss of perspective. The key activity is to start with the disease process or entering medical condition and not the end result (a negative outcome triggering a peer review). The SCA process then represents the disease or medical condition as all representative cases are in the denominator and the numerator can represent either successful or less successful care. PCR and APP PCPI processes do not have the capacity to do this. Therein is the data structure for competition.

The next step would be to link this activity with subsequent care/outcomes in the medical care continuum represented by the disease process. As an example, considering the hospital-based acute illness model, when the patient has been admitted, reviewing the linkage between the emergency medical care and the hospitalist care would be necessary. One example of this is the CVC life span audit in the subsequent section detailing completed audits. This audit broke the traditional lines of departmental care (activity only in the ED—placement of CVC) and discrete actions and instead focused on the patient movement and disease process during the admission and hospitalization. Despite the CVC placement being a discrete event in care, a properly leveled review can pull the event out of isolation and align departments through the cycle of managing the patient. Indeed, this is the reason the title of the audit was "CVC *life span*" as it represented the acute illness process and not the act of *placement*. As mentioned earlier, the entry trigger for any audit can be a discrete event but the properly focused or leveled audit process results in the value taken from the review. In a sense, the SCA process has potential to redirect even the medical culture within the institution as it aligns value of caring for the medical condition.

Admittedly, I am not so bold as to demand this as "the answer." But I would request the reader consider how the SCA process better meets the concepts Porter and Teisberg promote—a "step in the right direction."

■ FUNDAMENTALS OF CLINICAL AUDITING

Aspects of this method are embedded throughout the medical literature. One example, Mittiga depicts on the frequency of the procedures completed within a facility.[19] More recently, an article described the risk of serious events with repeated airway attempts.[20] Indeed, using the literature as a source for an auditing foundation is fundamental to the SCA process.

It is important to address the terms outcomes or processes and how they are used in this text. Outcomes are expected results from conserved processes or actions that heretofore have been described or defined through scientific evidence. Since we understand that the scientific literature that supports clinical practice is varied in its strength of association (observation to causation) we need to be selective in the use of literature as a basis for auditing clinical practice activities or processes. Based on the literature linked with each clinical entity, outcomes should be predictable when the practice is aligned with the literature recommendations (Figure 3-13). This does not discount that the patient has a spectrum of outcome expectations but necessarily has to address the technical outcomes associated with the disease presentation and focal physician actions.[21]

Donabedian states, "Outcomes … remain the ultimate validators of the effectiveness and quality of medical care." Yet he follows this statement with: "Another approach to assessment is to examine the process of care itself rather than its outcomes…. The estimates of quality that one obtains are less stable and less final than those that derive from the measurement of outcomes. They may … be more relevant to the question at hand: whether medicine is properly practiced."[22]

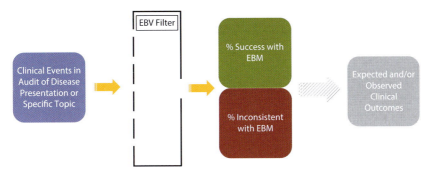

FIGURE 3-13. Relationship of auditing to expected clinical outcomes.

Largely clinical auditing is evaluating the processes or steps in care. There is a need to deconstruct macrometrics or outcomes such as survival or LOS into micrometrics or subprocesses in order to isolate, identify, impact, and improve. Afterward or concurrently we need to reconstruct all the processes and respect or represent the whole patient process.

■ PLANNING AN AUDIT (HOW TO CHOOSE A TOPIC)

This section is an attempt at proposing a comprehensive audit framework and the rationale for choices (Table 3-3). When I was initiating this program years ago, we focused on several articles in the literature that outlined the key malpractice events of our specialty. For emergency medicine this was missed myocardial infarction, missed appendicitis, missed ectopic pregnancy, missed fracture, missed FB, and other events of smaller frequency. Another approach would be to review the patterns or significant cases of the past several years of peer review events that your group has reviewed. A third approach could be polling the group and asking for audit topics based on disease presentations. This approach is especially beneficial as it initiates buy-in by the group members through early input, an ability to self-control or self-direct the process, as well as perhaps the best way of reflecting on the local pathology environment. An example of this would be to review ESRD patient management if the department had an increased number of dialysis patients due to that service-line presence. (By the by, focusing on differentiation is another aspect of Porter & Teisberg's "right" competition.) A fourth approach that

■ TABLE 3-3. Topic "Zones" for SCA

- Malpractice or risk presentations
- Peer review presentation
- Group input
- Literature as a specialty source

could be incorporated with the above approaches is the observation of the specialties' innovation (monitoring the specific literature for innovation that can be incorporated); one example including below is the incorporation of the ultrasound technique in CVC placement.

Looking at the assorted topics further, one could categorize these as high volume presentations, high-risk presentations, core measure topics, and "what we do as specific to our specialty" topics (Table 3-4). Many processes below have clinical policies or guidelines developed through ACEP or other agencies. Where appropriate it is valuable to incorporate the ACEP clinical polices as a baseline for a standard of emergency medicine practice (see politics). Probably the most "user-friendly" of guidelines are the Ottawa clinical decision rules as they combine safety, accuracy, and cost savings and can be easily incorporated into audit format.

Topics of audits:

- Cardiopulmonary arrest/resuscitation
  - Adult
  - Pediatric
  - Neonatal
- Abdominal pain/acute appendicitis (ACEP clinical policy)
- AMI/USA/CHF care (ACEP clinical policy)
- Shock/sepsis (Rivers article and Surviving Sepsis Campaign)
- Asthma/COPD care
- GIB intervention
- DKA treatment
- Meningitis evaluation/treatment
- Headache/SAH evaluation (ACEP clinical policy)
- Stroke intervention
- Seizure management (ACEP clinical policy)
- Overdose/suicide attempt (ACEP clinical policy)
- Anaphylaxis intervention
- Burn injuries and management

■ **TABLE 3-4.** Categories for SCA Topic Choice

- High-volume disease presentations
- High-risk disease presentations
- Core measure foci
- Specialty specific topics (EM = airway)
- Procedural
- Utilization
- Combination

- ED trauma resuscitation
- Ectopic pregnancy evaluation/resuscitation (ACEP clinical policy)
- Pediatric fever <3 months old
- Procedural sedation management (ACEP and AAP clinical policies)
- Hand/wrist injuries/bite wounds
- Dental pain/Rx
- Syncope (ACEP clinical policy and more)
- Ottawa clinical decision rules
- LLSA articles as sources

Based on the National Ambulatory Survey, abdominal pain or chest pain presentations are greater than 10% of ED volume annually.[23] The value in auditing these presentations, as mentioned before, is the combining of AMs and risk-related presentations. CP audits can be derivatives as well; STEMI, NSTEMI, CP in <40 years old, CP in the elderly, all can achieve comparative volumes. In abdominal pain, the disease presentations of ectopic pregnancy, appendicitis, PID, AAA can be included to manage risk. A third component could be procedural, including central venous catheter placement, intubations, lumbar punctures, suture repair of complex wounds. Combining the frequency of LPs with headache presentations could add value. Sepsis audits and ACLS management should be another critical audit as this type of care defines our specialty. Depending on the pediatric volume per ED facility, bronchiolitis, asthma, pharyngitis, and pediatric UTI are valuable audits, though a key management focus would be neonatal sepsis evaluation due to the high-risk nature of the presentation.

Finally, utilization can be incorporated into most audit cycles. For abdominal pain, the frequency of lipase testing, UA approach, and the use of urine cultures, as well as CT frequency in evaluations all can be incorporated.

■ DEVELOPING A COMPREHENSIVE AUDIT PLAN

Figure 3-14 shows a schematic of a year's worth of proposed audits for one emergency department from 2006. The audits were titled "Focused Review" and were quarterly (yellow bar). Note that this audit activity was in addition to the ongoing CAP and STEMI core measure work and the ongoing peer review (necessary as part of hospital/medical staff requirements). Figure 3-15 is a different plan over 3 years which describes the extent of foci that could be covered. With a goal of producing a quarterly audit, the previous audit's publication and "conversation" with the physicians is simultaneously occurring with the data collection of the subsequent (future) audit. Depending on the challenges of data collection and/or the challenges of communication and learning within each group, this framework or pace may not be achievable such that the audit pattern could be every 4 months or semiannually. It may also become more frequent over time. The goal would be to return to the disease presentation and review, potentially affirming xxxx Quality Committee Year: **2006-07**

Time Distributed Activity:

Activity	3	4	1	2
Quarter	3	4	1	2
Months	Oct-Dec	Jan-Mar	Apr-Jun	July-Sept
Focused Review	Report	Report	Report	Report
Indicator:	Peds Sepsis	Ddimer/PE	NSTEMI #2	Abscess/Cellulitis
SciHlth CAP/MI rpt	Ongoing			
Peer Review	Ongoing			
Utilization		Report		
Performance Analysis			Report	
CME	Report			
Other Projects:		Utilization Qtr	Procedure Activity Report	

FIGURE 3-14. Comprehensive annual audit plan (one group).

Year	Q1	Q2	Q3	Q4
1	AP - appendicitis	CP - low risk	Airway	Sepsis
2	Adult HA	ACLS	Neonatal Sepsis	CVC
3	NSTEMI	AP - pregnancy	PE/DVT	Adult UTI

FIGURE 3-15. Another schematic of a 3-year audit cycle.

successful intervention, reinforcing processes, and/or potentially incorporate new knowledge (Figure 3-16). This is a key difference with SCA to other hard methods of physician practice review. Peer review does not adequately monitor practice change. APP (Chapter 4) attempts this goal with the comparison pre- and postintervention but the volume of cases reviewed and the frequency as well as the lack of cycling is not adequate. Included in the following SCA examples is an audit on neonatal fever. The postintervention (second cycle) audit used the same data elements and showed significant practice change. This is the value of sequencing the audits and having a cycle that returns to disease topics.

■ DOING AN AUDIT

Once or as you are choosing the topic of the audit, a basic literature search is an important effort in order to frame the audit questions. Many times, you can rely on clinical policies, such as ACEP clinical policies or other such organizations (AHA) to pull out key components of the audit. It is important not to be too rigid or specific in your early framework, and to throw out a fairly wide net since these are observational studies. This is not an effort in producing a randomized controlled trial or a peer-reviewed journal article (see addendum). The goal is as described at the start, a reflective process, comparing site for individual practice with expected practice-based knowledge, and changing practice patterns.

Understandably, it is good to have some research background, but one does not have to know about ANOVA or hire a statistician. One needs to have an ability to manipulate data, controlling for and comparing variables, such that the audit data can mirror the literature source to the point that the populations are representative and comparison can occur. This adds legitimacy and validity to the clinical practice and constructive comparison with the potential for practice change becomes possible. In the subsequent published sepsis audit, the age range within the study population was consistent with the Rivers' study population. Determining that the local septic patient population was similar to the EBM and expected outcomes, physicians accepted the findings of their practice in comparison to the recommendations in the Surviving Sepsis Campaign.

Moreover, the goal is practice improvement such that local change is the focus. Percentage change in defined components within a time is often that desired outcome. One example of this is the neonatal audit in which the workup compliance (mostly LP completion) went from 68% to 96%.

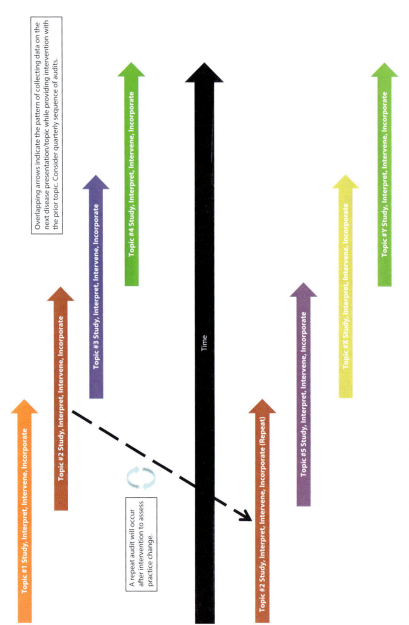

FIGURE 3-16. Audit cycle pattern: consider a macro-PDSA cycle.

■ **TABLE 3-5.** Study: Components of "Doing the Data"
1. Know your *good* EMR
2. Smart, cheap help
3. Basic statistics and programs
4. Time control—less data, more leadership
5. Use health system data sets

Study

Data collection has become easier as we know due to the electronic health records. There are several points for this section (Table 3-5). First, understand your EMR's capability, the tool may have some internal or embedded abilities to isolate data and make this easier to abstract. One example was the T system EV (no affiliation) in which we were able to isolate populations according to age, sex, chief complaint and this made the Neonatal Sepsis Audit very practical and efficient. As EMRs develop there will be increased search programming allowing for more robust clinical auditing. This will allow for a higher cycle frequency as well. Potentially the combination of multiple variables could be attained: consider the value of identifying pregnancy testing, timing of test, and patients with nonspecific abdominal pain presentations. Work on a more rapid identification of ectopic pregnancy could develop out of clinical auditing.

Second, hire some cheap but trainable help (a premed student, etc) to do your data collection! I was happy to write letters of recommendation, outlining the value of their work, in addition to paying an hourly rate.

Third, learn Microsoft's Excel, Access, and/or SPSS to enter and manipulate the data.

Fourth, stay simple, control a few variables, and spend much of your initial time setting up the practice comparison but reserving a large amount of your time for promoting, discussing, and interacting with your colleagues (be a cultural leader not just a data geek).

Fifth, other departments or organizations data sets can be obtained: the laboratory services (such as a list of patients tested for troponins and D-dimers), radiology services can provide lists of imaging types and patients, and the billing company can search and provide patient sets according to codes such as central-line placement or intubation. Real value on the audit comes with comparing or overlapping data sets.

Act

If one needs some background in statistics, etc, for data control, equally one needs political savvy, leadership technique and ability, and overall patience to advocate for practice change through the audit results. Groups that are engaged in clinical auditing (probably are not reading this book!), or at least have a robust, consistent, conserved peer review system, have already taken the big step of realizing continuous improvement is a necessary aspect of a healthy practice. They have decided that the capital "D" or "Dialogue" on how they practice is a group necessity. Considering *The Healthcare Quality Book*,[24] these are groups that are on the journey and are moving through Milestones 1, 2, and 3 (Chapter 5: Milestones in the Quality Measurement Journey). They have already realized that a stronger clinical practice has many benefits. In many ways, this "culture" could lead to the "responsiveness" described by Peter C. Wyer[25] (also discussed in the Knowledge Translation section below). In his discussion, he describes "responsiveness" as:

> the ability of such elements to adjust to and incorporate revisions in knowledge that call for revisions in practice...Responsiveness of a health measurement scale has been defined as "the ability of an instrument to measure a meaningful or clinically important change in a clinical state." Adapting this notion to KT, we may envision responsiveness as a measure of the extent to which clinically important changes in knowledge result in comparable changes in actions and recommendations on the part of caretakers, educators, and health care delivery systems. Corresponding incremental improvements in patient outcome are implicit in this notion.

In a comparison of the safety management in the nuclear energy industry, Pronovost and Hudson describe the benefit of group activity, "Local clinician led efforts that work through communities and change social norms are extremely effective, yet the most underdeveloped in health care. Communities of practice and quality improvement clinical communities are examples of local efforts that build relationships, network, learn and share, and have resulted in successful improvement efforts."[6] The strength of SCA is in its community or group approach with that group's willingness to be introspective.

Those groups who have not made this leap are in need of gentle encouragement and patience. Reflecting on this, the pace of auditing and switching disease or procedural topics must be slower. Often the pace of acceptance within a group can be assessed with intermittent questions of colleagues. Moreover, the slower pace encourages the "D" within groups and relieves any anxiety within the individual about oversight and job status/risk. Most importantly, the pace may allow for the learning and the clinical practice change to occur with deeper impact and retention.

■ PUBLISHING, POLITICS, AND PRACTICE CHANGE

Written communication is important, but it cannot be the sole method of relating these findings (Table 3-6). Communication methods should match the structure and functioning of the group: since EM physicians do not interact daily as a group but are shift working, electronic communication and/or print are forms that enable local communication. The audit summary should have an executive summary that is limited to one page, the first page, and a full audit summary is subsequent. The individual MD often will look at the executive summary and

■ **TABLE 3-6.** Actions After the Audit

Key: Patience

1. Publish the executive summary.
2. Publish the full audit.
3. Produce the leveled audit summaries depending on the audience.
4. Group presentation and discussion (attempt to sequence with production of summaries).
5. One-to-one discussions with MDs on individual data (both successful and inconsistent physician practice).
6. Follow-up or check-in with individual physicians.
7. Address operational process improvement identified within the audit.

then search for his/her individual data/scores. Often it is politically appropriate to create several audit summaries, one for the executive team that has identifiable individuals as well as possibly groups, and one for public review within the group, which is cleansed of identifiable individuals. This does not stop one's ability to have one-on-one conversations with individuals identified within the audit as needing improvement, but communication should be titrated to each level in order for education and acceptance. It is most important that the author control the copies that are produced that have individual physician identifiers as this information should only be observed within the group practice and not with hospital administration, nurse, staff, or administration or others associated with the institution or health care. This cannot be overemphasized. The lack of control of the data summary and conclusions could undermine the whole clinical performance improvement program which works on trust.

A typical sequence of intervention is the publishing of the audit summary, the group presentation, followed by the one-on-one conversation(s). Again the remarkable aspect of auditing in comparison to peer review is that the publishing of the audit and the group presentation of data allows for a multilevel approach to learning.

It is my personal opinion (and those of others) that a multilevel intervention works best when providing feedback to physicians.[26] Many physicians look to the audit summaries as affirmation of their work; indeed most often the outcome is such a positive reinforcement of care with additional minor considerations that can fine-tune the practice. Many physicians appear to learn and modify their practice simply from the knowledge that auditing is occurring (Hawthorne effect) or through the individual review of the audit summary (perhaps learning from others' [anonymous] "challenges" without any group or individual conversations).

Often prior to having one-on-one conversations, a group presentation well sets the tone of the review. As mentioned earlier, physicians are keenly objective and will attend to the presented data. Allowing for criticism of the data in a public forum is ego-challenging for the auditor but, placed in the context of larger goals, allows for a heightened, ongoing interest by the physicians/group. It also improves the future audit approach and data value via suggestions and sets the tone of the "D" (dialogue) culture in which the auditor is subjecting him/herself to the group in addition to mutual ownership of the outcomes ("we are all in this together").

The one-on-one conversations with physicians deemed needing a conversation are a necessary component of the audit process. Often these physicians are selected based on a postdetermined cutoff after reviewing the data or based on an outstanding aspect after comparing the individual data with the group outcomes. Several simple suggestions will hopefully result in a good conversation. First, it is helpful that the physician leadership publically advocate and support the auditor role; second, the auditor has to be a physician in order to approach a physician about his/her practice; third, recognize the deeply personal commitment that every physician has to quality of patient care (even if he/she cannot fully define what that is for every individual case—they know it/feel it—the auditor's job is to define it); fourth, (similar to the peer review discussion on feedback) choose a good time and neutral place—not after a night shift and not before a shift, allowing the receiving physician some determination and be patient if there is a time delay (the goal is listening to your information and suggestions); fifth, present the "challenges" in the background of the group and the literature to avoid isolated interpretation as in single-case peer review; sixth, finish with a conversation about improvement and allow for the physician to suggest methods of intervention and/or make suggestions for positive change. It would be valuable to create a check-in point in the future to reinforce the learning and agreed upon goals; the knowledge of the repeated audit and comparison is a natural pressure for practice change.

The more the auditor practices this, the easier it becomes (including that the group and individual physicians become more comfortable with the conversations). Moreover, it is always healthy to have some conversations with physicians who had high success with certain audits. This effort has much positivity: mental health for the auditor, affirmation of that physician's practice, and advocacy of the fairness and overall goals of the SCA process.

In addition, during several clinical audits, we identified operational conflicts that impacted clinical quality. There is a surprising benefit to addressing the operational conflict identified within the audits. This allowed for physicians to have more acceptance of the data and the recommendations about his or her clinical practice. This again was a reinforcement of the philosophy of improvement that processes and not individuals are often causes of defects. It was an interesting observation that addressing these processes resulted in gaining ground culturally.

■ THE OBSERVED PATTERNS OF PRACTICE

Unique to SCA is the granularity and the breadth of the data reviewed. The randomness and infrequency of PCR cannot properly represent a physician or a group practice. A properly constructed clinical audit can represent the decision making or management patterns of each physician. This granularity can allow for comparison to the evidence or science related to the decisions or clinical management and thereby allowing for specific directed feedback to each physician and potentially in general to the group.

The physician practice patterns observed during audits can be categorized according to (1) consistency with patients and (2) alignment with the evidence. The first category is random practice activity without apparent alignment (Figure 3-17A). In this category, the physician has no pattern of practice on managing a series of similar presentations. The practice at times is consistent with the literature but other patients are inconsistently managed within the literature recommendations. An example of this irregular practice was observed in the double audit of neonatal sepsis in which several physicians were randomly, inconsistently completing a lumbar puncture procedure (LP) despite the same age, fever presentation, and advocacy of the guideline. Some pediatric patients had LPs completed whereas others did not; there was no apparent pattern. In the extreme, the pattern of practice could be consistent but dramatically outside of the literature directive (Figure 3-17B, C). Several physicians in the D-dimer and CT utilization audit ordered zero CT angiograms despite a range of D-dimer and Wells scores that based on probability and the literature would have supported an imaging study or, conversely, ordered CT angiogram studies on 100% of patients regardless of Wells scores or D-dimer results. Both these patterns could represent incomplete medical decision making and thus risk, either the excessive radiation of overimaging potentially out of concern for missed diagnosis and forfeiting the supportive literature that ensures practice safety or the simplifying of practice in a negation of disease prevalence. Unfortunately these unusual patterns could put the next patient at risk as well as having the potential to compromise operations and flow.

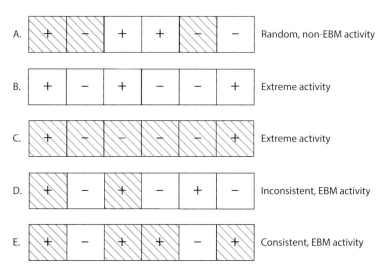

FIGURE 3-17. Observed patterns of practice (shaded is activity; +/− represents EBM support of activity).

In my experience, the above physicians who show distinctly irregular technical patterns will show this in sequential audits. The auditor and the aware, nonpunitive group need to support these physicians in efforts to renew and redirect them back into technical high quality. The value of the SCA method with its breadth and granularity allows the auditor and group to visualize whether there are distinct knowledge and medical decision-making gaps in an individual's practice or that this is a global practice problem.

The second category is a conserved activity but the activity may have some inconsistencies with the literature (Figure 3-17D). In this category, the physician is consistent with decision making and activity and the clinical practice is irregularly aligned with EBM descriptions. One example of this pattern is also from the double audit of neonatal sepsis in which a physician was consistent and complete with the evaluation including a lumbar puncture and blood cultures and consistent with providing ampicillin and gentamicin rather than ampicillin and cefotaxime/ceftriaxone. Understandably this physician is practicing more consistently with the evidence and a minor adjustment in practice after identifying gaps in knowledge or decision making could be the conversation between the physician and the auditor. Interestingly, the author will forward that the outcome of the conversation or dialogue may not be directive; the physician may have good justification for his or her decision based on experience and locality and is attempting to bridge the evidence with experience. This should lead to a larger group discussion and the weighing of practice differences toward agreement. Still, considering the goal of reducing variability the single physician more likely would amend decision making and practice pattern toward the group pattern (as long as the group pattern represented EBM). The value of this change is evident when observing the nursing practice in which consistency and patterns in operations are valued. A single, infrequent gentamicin dose in comparison to cephalosporin administration can cause delays in care and patient risk. Intervening with this physician should be much easier than the above random practice in which the auditor can applaud the consistency and suggest a minor change to practice which again may be easier to accept. Moreover, a group presentation and discussion may realign this physician once he or she is more aware of the evidence/literature well ahead of the one-on-one conversation (next section).

The third category is the conserved, evidence-based practice (Figure 3-17E). This is the physician who appears to have determined a course of activity with the specific clinical presentation, is well aware of the specific evidence relating to the disease process and management, and is consistently performing within those rules. Examples of these physicians are apparent within several audits in this text. In the D-dimer and CT utilization audit many physicians were either consistent employing the Wells criteria and D-dimer levels to decide on which patients to obtain CT angiograms. Likewise, several physicians were consistent with the Chest Pain Audit in which they determined the low-risk patient with a single negative troponin was deemed reasonable to exclude acute coronary syndrome. Notably, these consistent practices allow for operational efficiency and high-quality, safe care. As mentioned subsequently, an affirmation of practice is invaluable and absolutely necessary when auditing and determining consistency and high accuracy. Physicians will take personal pride in their practice audit results and recognize the alignment with EBM sources during the discussion.

As expected, bundling individual practice patterns to represent a group practice will result in a heterogeneous presentation. This could be viewed in regard to one disease process or audit of such or several audits could be combined and a "genotype" of the practice could be created. The value of the genotype view is to identify the gaps in knowledge and technique that could require a focused intervention. These areas could be organ system or condition specific, pulmonary management including COPD, pediatric asthma, and pulmonary emboli management. It may be that a group would show high consistency and accuracy with EB recommendations in cardiac disease including HTN management but have gaps in orthopedic management. An example is in the subsequent audits with the recognition (and intervention) of a lack of ultrasound-guided central venous catheter placement. Though the author initiated the audit having become aware of the EM literature and CLABSI discussion, the gap in knowledge and technique was confirmed with an audit and was present within the practices of many physicians and not rare physician deficits. Group intervention ensued. As mentioned in the Introduction section, all physicians have weaknesses or gaps in practice but many have similar gaps. Identifying the gaps leads to the group dialogue on how to practice and a determination of practice direction and consistency within the locality. Based on the genotype or audit results, imagine a "reading of the code," intervention could be largely directed at individuals and less at the group, whereas it could be wholly a group process (all the individual physicians). Specifically addressing technical gaps within individuals and the group would alter the genotype and "phenotype" (Figure 3-18). As discussed further in Chapter 5, this activity has the potential to determine a group's branding or phenotype as well.

■ AUDIT CYCLE FREQUENCY AS PERTAINING TO PHYSICIAN TECHNICAL DECAY

There are many options and approaches as well as disease foci to create a sequential clinical audit format. I have provided a long list and some general decision-making framework for selecting the audit topic, categories such as malpractice risk, peer review triggers, group interest, local disease prevalence, high-volume issues, and specialty-specific topics.

We know practice atrophies over time.[27] The initial audit goal is a description of the individual and group technical status, identifying the gaps between EBM expectations and actual practice. The goal of repeated cycles of the same audit is to determine closure of the practice gap, elevation of generalized technical quality within the individual and group, introduction and monitoring of new knowledge (KT), and also for monitoring technical decay. These latent goals emphasize the change in quality of care over time. Questions then arise: How often should the repeat audit be? In what time frame? Can the frequency be representative?

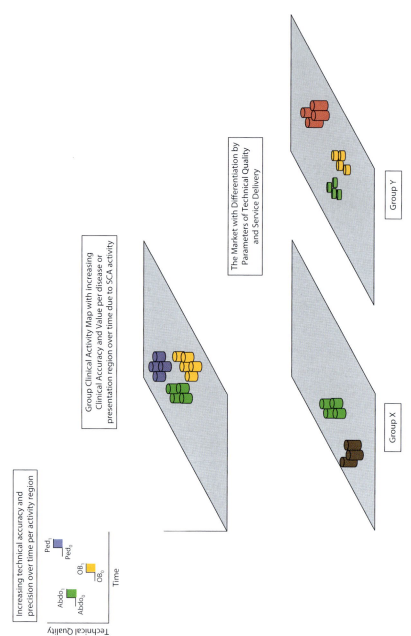

FIGURE 3-18. Bundled audits representing group practice.

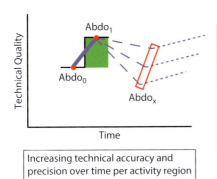

Clinical Auditing determined technical quality at $Abdo_0$ and at $Abdo_1$ with the blue line representing the learning part of the experience curve. The dashed blue lines represent examples of 3 potential decay patterns over time ($Abdo_1$-$Abdo_2$ states). Subsequent interventions and clinical audits (at point $Abdo_x$) may cause upturn within curve (dotted lines).

Increasing technical accuracy and precision over time per activity region

FIGURE 3-19. Example of experience curve for abdominal presentation focus.

Pusic et al. discuss experience curves in relationship to emergency medicine learning and simulation tools.[28] Within the article the authors describe experience curves as "combinations of learning and forgetting curves that can demonstrate a single, longitudinal representation of knowledge and skill acquisition and decay over time." Indeed, the reader can image this curve as a saw tooth pattern with upslope representing intervention and learning and the downslope representing forgetting and knowledge or skill decay (Figure 3-19). The authors note that some emergency physicians will continue to have increasing learning and performance over time through deliberate increased effort as such; other physicians will plateau but not have decay, and still other physicians will have decay in performance. Decay can be globally present or more likely specific to the knowledge or skill. Factors that contribute to decay of knowledge or skill are the nature of the knowledge or skill (increased decay rate with higher complexity), infrequent practice exposure (less exposure with higher decay rate), as well as the strength and pattern of initial training (decreasing decay). An emergency medicine practice could then be dynamically viewed as a collection or bundling of experience curves at different stages of decay related to disease topics or procedural foci. In this view, gaps in technical quality become evident. Considering this model, the audit cycle frequency may have to be variable based on the specific topic and the determined level of acceptable competency associated with the knowledge and the skill. This model can be contrasted with the 5- or 10-year cycle to determine public competency of practice (MOC).

Unfortunately, there is a lack of literature describing the patterns of skill or knowledge decay over time for breadth of pathology the emergency physician must manage and thus directing the frequency of a cycle on a specific topic or disease presentation is challenging to estimate. Several interesting EM articles reinforce the above model as well as the need for auditing.

Recognizing the infrequency of prehospital pediatric airway compromise and the need for ongoing EMS training, Youngquist et al. evaluated paramedic efficacy with RSI and BVM techniques and concluded that the pediatric airway management skill performance decreased significantly over 6 months after training.[29]

Thus, the study authors discovered a decay rate for their population as well as defined a competency threshold. The authors also identified a gap between self-efficacy and skill retention in which paramedics maintained confidence in management despite evidence of incorrect skill performance. This study uniquely advances the idea that reliance on physicians'/providers' self-determination when their technical skills are waning may not be advantageous. Some skills or practice technical aspects may need high-frequency intervention regardless of provider self-assessment due to the risk and high-valued management. In emergency medicine, airway management would be such as skill. The findings of no correlation between self-assessment and technical skill competency reinforce the argument for more aggressive, beyond peer review and passive CME, methods of maintaining technical quality in emergency medicine.

Intervention, though varied in form, can be effective in maintaining technical quality. Kovacs et al. studied airway management in medical students, evaluating the rate of skill decay after an initial education program.[30] In comparison to a nonrefresher training control, the interventional group received eight subsequent sessions of airway practice and scenarios over 10 months. Despite continued technical decay, the knowledge and skill decay rate was reduced in the interventional group. In both groups decay was apparent at the first assessment (16 weeks) after initial training. This study supports an audit frequency as well as a successful intervention method.

Contrasting Kovacs' study, Su et al. noted a loss of paramedic resuscitation knowledge within 12 months of a PALS course and also concluded that the 6-month interventions (repeat examination and mock resuscitation) were not successful at limiting decay.[31] The authors also provide an excellent review of other ACLS activities and assessment of knowledge decay mentioning that postintervention decay has been observed within 2 weeks, 5, 6, and 12 months dependent on the study. This text will not address various educational interventions other than to agree with the authors that decay may vary dependent on type of intervention.

One clinical audit example, the Central Venous Catheter Audit in this chapter of the book, I promoted a threshold number of annual central venous catheter placements that could represent ongoing competence or trigger necessary review/mediation. This threshold attempted to represent a complication rate and threshold of competency and could be complementary to the individual physician data and singular procedural outcomes. This concept represents the Pusic decay model of learning and forgetting and is fairly novel, though rudimentary, in monitoring physician technical competency in which a competency level and decay rate could be established.

Operationally a local SCA program could be structured in relationship to the focal disease processes and the known (discovered) decay rates (both native and interventional-adjusted). The sequential audits would further define the focal experience curve and interventions could be efficiently applied. It should be noted that clinical auditing is both an analytical/tracking process and an intervention. The activity of technical gap exposure, provision of this knowledge to participants combined with other interventions, and the group dialogue results in practice change. In my experience, audit (including feedback) alone has interventional effect.[32] One could also argue that ongoing practice is intervention; a lack of exposure is known to cause knowledge or skill decay. Yet experience without a comparison may be inadequate to ensure higher technical quality. Again, the clinical auditing program promotes comparison of practice actions to EBM such that the physician maintains a status on the experience curve above the competency level and this experience curve is maximally aligned with EBM and expected outcomes associated with high technical quality.

In combining the discussion on practice pattern observed within the audits in this section, it may be reasonable to project that the observed practice pattern variation may be related to the knowledge or skill decay and the physician's technical quality point on the experience curve. A physician practice pattern in alignment with EBM may be on the learning curve above the competency threshold, either ascending due to recent individual education/intervention or clinical exposure or descending (Figure 3-17E). Equally, physician patterns outside the EBM criteria may represent the forgetting curve (Figure 3-17A-C).

In conclusion, the auditor may have to consider the state of the audit program in determining an audit frequency. Early in the program, in acknowledgment of the introduction and physician consideration/participation in the new program, the audit pattern may be a fixed 3- to 4-month frequency in which the individual and group's practice patterns can be described. With a developed program, the frequency of audits can become dependent on the above discussion and related to specific topic experience curves.

◼ COMMENT ON KNOWLEDGE TRANSLATION, CME, AND SEQUENTIAL CLINICAL AUDITING

SCA is knowledge translation (KT) and CME. A definition of KT is any activity or process that facilitates the transfer of high-quality evidence from research into effective changes in health policy, practice, or products.[33] This definition well incorporates the SCA process based on (1) SCA's inherent structure of identifying practice gaps between evidence and predicted outcomes and current practice and (2) its method of changing practice pattern through its topic focus and associated evidential support, effort to mediate the value of experience with EBM, and direct intervention on an individual, group, and organizational level that extends beyond individual decision making impacting an environment for EB practice.[34]

KT must be viewed in the heterogeneous landscape of knowledge acquirement, retention, and gap pattern within physician practice. Relating the prior discussion on experience curves while describing the knowledge and application gap differences can be realized. New evidence uptake as an EM resident without prior knowledge and experience could be different learning from the experienced physician in which the former has no decay aspect of an experience curve whereas the latter may have learning, decay, and relearning curves. Even a third process of learning may be involved with the experienced physician in which there is no decay or forgetting curve but an evolution of knowledge requires a replacement of facts and potentially a forced forgetting or unlearning for new knowledge. Thus in relation to the above mentioned gap in KT, the vision of the gap must be dynamic, not static, and that the state of knowledge is a dynamic balance between learning and forgetting as well as the replacement of newer knowledge. Unfortunately this book cannot extend further into issues of learning theory. Notably, the SCA process can represent this dynamic landscape as evident in the discussion on patterns of practice which could represent the variety of gaps present within physicians and groups.

Graham et al. introduced a knowledge-to-action map emphasizing the theory of KT.[35] As with many improvement efforts, the components of the map are consistent with a PDSA cycle and as has been described, SCA is a macro-PDSA format. Components of the map follow: initially a problem must be identified—this being the gap in EBM expected practice and observed practice. The knowledge associated with the activity would then be reviewed for value in the setting and adapted to the local environment. Interventions are implemented including the acknowledgment of the gap, the individual practice patterns compared with potentially more valued patterns. Further auditing would monitor the sustained use of the EB knowledge within the practice as well as monitor selected outcomes associated with the EB literature.

In their article on the development of the consensus conference, Lang et al. describe a model of KT in which a hierarchical pyramid of evidence based on increasing strength and applicability can be funneled into an application pipeline.[33] As advocated in this text, the ACEP clinical policies can represent this higher level of evidence and applicability. Grimshaw et al. concur in their discussion, indicating that "up-to-date systemic reviews or other syntheses of global evidence" should be the "basic unit of knowledge translation."[34] Though the SAEM conference model identifies the variable strength of evidence for application, the SCA process recognizes the complexities of application including the transparent group process valuing auditing of practice, choice of focus, and commitment to ongoing dialogue which helps mediate the incorporation of new or different evidence into the experiential realm. Depending on the group's consideration of value, varying levels of EB literature, experiences of the local environment and community values may be incorporated: consider the *seizure audit* in which the management of a motor vehicle license was observed in comparison to the use of the Wells criteria for the assessment of PE risk. The former has community value and minimal science in comparison to the latter.

As above, the group culture (representing the combination of individual states of acceptance) has a significant impact on practice change. In this text, I have described it as the group dialogue about the quality of practice promoted in the brand. Peter Wyer proposes a quality indicator of the KT process as "responsiveness" of elements to adjust to and incorporate revisions in knowledge that call for revisions in practice.[25] Though the responsiveness is intended to represent elements such as research, education, etc, this description well includes the physician culture and group dialogue that is essential for practice change and an effective audit program. Essentially, I have promoted the SCA as a medium that represents functional, "responsive" group culture.

Grimshaw and colleagues break down the KT process into further components reflecting on the choice of knowledge forms (systemic reviews as above), the qualities of the messenger, the recognition of the variability of and within audiences, the barriers to KT, and the choice of interventions.[34] As has been described in this this chapter and in Chapter 5, the SCA method incorporates much of this discussion and fits their description of a "tailored intervention" composing many aspects of more valued intervention.

Specifically, Grimshaw et al. describe the messenger as having to have credibility. An authoritative physician or physician organization and its endorsement of the subject matter can influence receiving physician acceptance. Indeed, the internal candidate for this activity should be recognized by peers as clinically solid, though I would advocate that not only should the individual be technically solid but a stronger position would be as a colleague who also mediates the process for the group but is part of the group and not external to it. Again, the latter position may be a goal and pragmatically to initiate a program may involve the more technically accurate physician.

As for choosing interventions, Grimshaw and colleagues provide a review of the literature on effective KT interventions and this can be compared to the SCA model. Of the effective interventions described, the description of SCA incorporates (1) printed education materials including the distribution of clinical policies, guidelines, or pertinent articles for physician review and education; (2) the summaries of audits are written and distributed to individuals and groups as a form of "persuasive communication," impactful with data and acknowledgment of practice; (3) education beyond individual communication involves interactive workshops and departmental meetings encouraging group discussion, reflection on local standards, and criticism of the audit process; (4) the auditors should "tailor their approach to the characteristics of the individual health care provider" understanding that acceptance and reflection vary per person; and (5) beyond the previously mentioned messenger, other physicians may represent local opinion leaders and can be "educationally influential" such as a physician subspecialized in ultrasound or another technical who then can be a strong advocate and resource for practice change.

Considering the direct comparison of practice and the literature, the SCA is more impactful when compared to the passive absorption of lectures or readings which is currently the predominant form of CME.[36] The difficulty is in the form; externally developed and passive CME is unable to be selective enough to identify individual physician needs but is reliant on (or ignorant of) the individual physician in determining his or her needs. Unfortunately, as this text has discussed, the physician/provider often cannot determine his or her individual gaps or rate of knowledge and skill decay. Instead, a smorgasbord of offerings and a smothering of material are directed at the physician; most of which (from personal experience) are not absorbed. SCA is CME but more specific to the local group. SCA is able to identify the unique, discrete gaps in technical quality, experience, and knowledge decay, and incorporate effective, timely interventions. Moreover, SCA is a better method of incorporating new knowledge specific to the local need.

A CONSIDERATION OF SAMPLING SIZE

One of the main criticisms of the current methods of physician practice review is the infrequent, low-volume patient care or chart review. Considering this as a sampling issue, a question could be asked, "What would be a necessary sample size that could represent the physician's annual practice?"

The challenge with emergency medicine and with most general medicine is the heterogeneity of disease presentations that represent the "practice." Thus audits must achieve high value, not just volume but a breadth of presentation to ensure the goal of a comprehensive review.

Statistically, sequential clinical auditing is simply nonprobability sampling and the convenience samples have all the inherent biases.[37] Due to the EMR, it was feasible to include all subjects as consecutive samples.[38] Reviewing the published audits in this chapter, the Central Venous Catheter Audit had 233 cases—patients over 1 year and the Double Audit of Neonatal Sepsis Practice Compliance Guideline for Fever in the Less Than 60-Day-Old Audit covered all the febrile neonatal presentations in the system for 1 year.

Moreover, the goal of SCA is clinical review and a comparison of practice to outcomes. This addresses care delivery and is an effort in "improving process of care."[39] This is not "improving clinical evidence" or basic research and the tools of these approaches are often different. In short to consider the "power" of the study is to misclassify the goal and methods of the SCA. Consistent with the goal of improving care process, the clinical practice findings had associated learning through comparison and this allowed for practice change.

Can you then have an operational goal for representation? Would 10% of annual practice be attainable? Considering an FT EM physician may see 2000 patients annually, would a sequence of audits review 200 patients per physician? The answer depends on the foci of the audits, whether the disease or condition frequency is high and whether mechanistically the data can be abstracted well. Still, it is not just the numbers but the value gained from the audit. Considering the Double Audit of Neonatal Sepsis Practice Compliance Guideline for Fever in the Less Than 60-Day-Old Audit (given below), most physicians had only one case but the collective learning within the group in regard to the sample was invaluable as seen by the follow-up audit showing practice change.

EXAMPLES OF CLINICAL AUDITS

In the following audit example section, there are several references to similar published, peer-reviewed studies. None of the audit examples in this primer have been published or peer reviewed in a formal publication manner; the reasoning is that this work was local and internal, regarded as peer review and under legal protection as quality improvement such that some findings might be admissible if published. The author's goal was to improve the local environment first and subsequently advise the larger community. The mentioning of similar published studies to the following audits is the author's effort to assure you, the reader, that he knew what he was doing (humor). Please also recognize that many of the audits predated the published articles (ego).

Every effort was made to make the sites of review anonymous. If an EMR name is mentioned, it is due to the specific use of the tool and not due to any affiliation with the product or corporation (the author has completed audits on many EMR products but will not divulge his favorites). Several audits in this text have been minimally modified from the originals due to need for text structure and for anonymity.

I describe (italics) some of the nuances, challenges, or interesting outcomes from each study is at the start of each audit summary.

CHEST PAIN AUDIT

Patients, Aged 24-39 Years Old, Presenting With Chest Pain

Author's Comments

The patient with chest pain is one of the more frequent ED presentations. Due to this volume and frequency, actions taken in the evaluation have the potential to compromise ED flow. Often protocols, especially those initiated in triage and prior to MD evaluation, are insensitive to age and risk factors yet as per Marsan article, the potential to stratify these patients and minimize risk, work, and cost and still achieve good outcomes is present.[40] *As an entry clinical audit the low-risk CP entity may be valuable to initiate the conversation of practice variance and/or the consideration of protocol review/revision within the physician group. Many systems have developed observational units to manage these patients and attach various types of additional studies as well as monitoring. Efficiency and throughput of these units are important and the consideration of controlling entry variability is a method to heighten observational unit management. Most notable through this audit is that the type and quality of entry determines efficiency in the unit as much as what is done during the unit evaluation.*

This is a simple audit that is based on one article but directly exposes practice variance between physicians. The potential for modifying triage-driven protocols and/or entry criteria to observation units would assist heightened physician awareness. Hard copy protocols and checklists will reinforce culture/practice change. Reaudit in 6 months considering volume. These data were granular to the level of individual physicians and group discussion as well as individual conversations is possible.

I end this audit in a conversational mode as this was the first or introductory audit and view of this group's clinical activity I wanted to softly sell the findings. Clearly there was great variability in practice approach in a group that touted clinical strength.

Background

Marsan et al. in "Evaluation of a Clinical Decision Rule for Young Adult Patients with Chest Pain"[40] combined a clinical decision rule for adults younger than 40 years of age with chest pain (no known cardiac history and either no classic cardiac risk factors or a normal ECG indicating low risk) and a negative set of cardiac markers at the time of ED presentation would reduce the risk of 30-day adverse CV events, AMI, and ACS to <0.2%. They concluded that this decision rule could be used to limit unnecessary hospital evaluations and admissions.

This is an observational study replicating the Marsan et al. article methods on a convenience sample of patients in order to observe the clinical activity and medical decision making according to this population.

Methods

Using the EMR system and selecting for "Reports" then selecting "ED Active Patients Log" determined the active patients who presented to the ED during the 1-month time window. Further categorization was determined using chest pain as the chief complaint. Note: Chest pain as the main complaint had to be confirmed in the provider's note otherwise the case was be excluded (four cases). Age range was then selected for 24-39 years, this being consistent with the definition of a low-risk population in the Marsan et al. article.

Data abstraction included the cardiovascular risk factors (noted with low case key letter): HTN (h), DM (d), known CAD (c), history of MI (m), CABG (s), CHF (f), CRI/ESRD (r), and cocaine usage. No mention of drug abuse in the social history was determined as a negative for cocaine use. ECG interpretation was primarily based on the ED provider's notation and secondarily on the computer interpretation when ED provider note was absent; all negatives were interpreted as a normal ECG. Any abnormality (nonspecific T waves, STD, etc) was interpreted as an abnormal ECG.

Outcomes were determined from the discharge report on all admitted patients. Thirty-day outcomes were limited to an inspection of the medical record.

Results (Table 3-7)

Sixty-one cases were reviewed for this one month. Forty-four patients were female (72%); 39 patients were triaged ESI 3 (64%); and 20 patients were triaged ESI 2 (33%). Thirty providers were reviewed; providers had seen between one to six patients (mode = 1).

Average LOS was 6.83 hours (1.5-28.25 hours). Ten patients (16%) were admitted; six to CDU, four to inpatient status. Of the 10 admissions, one provider had two admissions with a single admission for eight physicians, respectively. The provider with the two admissions placed both in CDU.

Thirty-nine patients had no CVD history (64%). Twenty-two patients had cardiac risk factors: 13 with hypertension only, 9 with hypertension and either diabetes, CHF hx, and/or renal disease.

No patient was identified as using cocaine.

■ TABLE 3-7. Low-Risk CP Presentation and Disposition, Observation Unit Efficiency

DOS	Prov	LOS	ESI	Disp	MRN	CVD hx (y/n)	Type CVD	Coc (y/n)	ECG nml (y/n)	Trop # If Done	Second Trop?	Trop Time ▲	Return in 30 Days?	Outcome	If Admit Outcome?
11/1	A	5.75	2			y	h, m, f	n	n	0.03			n		
11/2	P	5.00	3			y	h	n	y	0.01			n		
11/2	M	4.50	2			y	h	n	y	0.01	0.01	1.5	n		
11/4	O	21.50	3	CDU		y	h, d	n	n	0.04			n		nml cath
11/4	S	28.25	3			n		n	y	0.01	0.01	4	n		
11/5	S	11.50	3	CDU		y	h	n	y	0.01	0.01	3	n		No study
11/5	H	2.50	3			n		n	y	0.01			y	Not 4 CP	
11/6	A	3.50	3			n		n	n	0.01			n		
11/7	C	2.50	3			y	h	n	y	na			n		
11/7	M	7.50	3			n		n	y	na			n		
11/6	R	4.00	3			y	h	n	n	na			n		
11/1	A	5.33	2			n		n	y	0.01			n		
11/6	M	5.25	3			n		n	n	na			n		
11/1	K	5.75	2			n		n	y	na			y	SCC	
11/9	B	6.00	3			n		n	y	0.01			n		
11/9	L	5.00	2	INPT		y	h, d, r	n	y	0.01			n		No study
11/10	H	9.00	2			n		n	y	0.01			n		
11/11	M	10.50	2			y	h	n	n	0.02	0.01	5	n		
11/11	M	4.00	3			n		n	n	na			n		

(Continued)

■ **TABLE 3-7.** Low-Risk CP Presentation and Disposition, Observation Unit Efficiency (*Continued*)

DOS	Prov	LOS	ESI	Disp	MRN	CVD hx (y/n)	Type CVD	Coc (y/n)	ECG nml (y/n)	Trop # If Done	Second Trop?	Trop Time ▲	Return in 30 Days?	Outcome	If Admit, Outcome?
11/12	S	8.00	3	CDU		y	h	n	n	0.01	0.01	3	n		Neg PET
11/13	N	2.00	4			n		n	n	na			n		
11/13	S	3.75	3			n		n	y	na			y	Dx GERD	
11/12	A	5.00	3			n		n	na	na			n		
11/12	A	6.00	3			n		n	n	0.01			n		
11/10	C	5.75	2			y	h	n	n	0.01			n		
11/8	L	6.50	3			n		n	y	na			n		
11/10	P	25.00	3	CDU		y	h	n	n	0.01	0.01	3	n		sECHO neg
11/10	N	5.50	3			n		n	y	0.01			n		
11/9	S	4.75	3			n		n	na	na			n		
11/9	S	4.25	2			n		n	n	0.01			n		
11/17	S	4.75	2			n		n	na	na			n		
11/18	O	6	2			y	h, d, r	n	n	0.01	0.01	3.5	n		
11/18	D	4.5	3			n		n	y	na			n		
11/19	D	7	3			n		n	y	na			n		
11/19	S	3.75	2	INPT		y	h, r, f	n	n	0.14			n		No study
11/19	S	8	3	CDU		n		n	y	0.01	0.01	3	n		No study
11/19	R	3.5	2			n		n	y	0.01			n		

11/19	R	4	2		n		n	y	0.01	0.01		n	
11/20	O	3	3		n		n	y	na			n	
11/20	N	1.5	3		n		n	y	na			n	
11/21	N	4.5	3		n		n	y	0.01	0.01		n	
11/22	R	3.5	3	INPT	y	h, r	n	n	0.04	0.04	2	n	Neg PET
11/22	M	6.75	2		y	h, d	n	n	0.01	0.04	14	n	
11/23	S	2	3		n		n	y	0.01			n	
11/27	N	17.75	3		n		n	n	0.01			n	
11/28	N	6.5	1	INPT	y	h, r, f, d	n	n	0.1	0.12	3	y	CHF exac
11/28	S	9.75	3		y	h	n	y	0.01			n	
11/29	S	5.75	2		y	h, d, f	n	y	0.03			n	
11/29	B	5	2		n		n	y	0.01			n	
11/29	S	4.5	3		n		n	y	0.01			n	
11/30	N	2	3		n		n	y	na			n	
11/20	B	10.5	3		n		n	y	na			y	CP non cad
11/22	R	4.25	3		n		n	y	0.01			n	
11/26	B	13.75	3		n		n	y	0.01			y	Leg pain
11/28	R	4.5	3		n		n	y	na			n	
11/17	N	16.5	2	CDU	y	d	n	n	0.01	0.01	2	y	No study
11/26	C	7.25	3		n		n	y	0.01			n	

(Continued)

■ TABLE 3-7. Low-Risk CP Presentation and Disposition, Observation Unit Efficiency *(Continued)*

DOS	Prov	LOS	ESI	Disp	MRN	CVD hx (y/n)	Type CVD	Coc (y/n)	ECG nml (y/n)	Trop # If Done	Second Trop?	Trop Time ▲	Return in 30 Days?	Outcome	If Admit, Outcome?
11/19	A	4.75	2			n		n	y	na			y	ha	
11/29	B	6.5	3			n		n	y	0.01			n		
11/18	B	3.75	3			y	h	n	y	0.01			n		
11/16	B	7	2			y	d	n	y	0.01			n		

DOS = date of service
Prov = provider
LOS = length of stay
ESI = emergency severity index
Disp = disposition
MRN = medical record number
CVD hx = cardiovascular disease history
CVD = cardiovascular disease
Coc = cocaine usage history
ECG = electrocardiogram
Trop = troponin level
CDU = clinical decision unit
INPT = inpatient admission
HTN (h), DM (d), known CAD (c), history of MI (m), CABG (s), CHF (f), CRI/ESRD (r)
SCC = sickle cell crisis
GERD = gastroesophageal reflux disease
PET = positron emission tomography test
ECHO = echocardiogram

Low-Risk Group (Figure 3-20)

- Twenty-nine patients met the low-risk criteria; negative CVD history, no cocaine usage, and a normal ECG.
- Twelve patients were discharged without a troponin level.
- Fourteen patients had a single troponin level (all negative) and were discharged (48%). *Complete low-risk pattern.*
- Two patients had a second troponin level (both negative) and were discharged.
- One patient was admitted to the CDU (and had two troponin levels (negative) and no study).
- Six of 29 patients returned within 30 days of initial evaluation for issues unrelated to CVD. None were admitted.

High-Risk Group

- Twenty-two patients did not meet the low-risk criteria due to positive CVD risk factors/history and 10 patients did not meet low-risk criteria based on abnormal ECG (7) or no ECG done (3).

High-Risk due to CVD History (Figure 3-21)

- Two patients were discharged without troponin levels.
- Twenty patients had at least one troponin level (two were positive).
- Eleven patients had one troponin level; three patients were admitted one with a positive troponin level; eight patients were discharged.

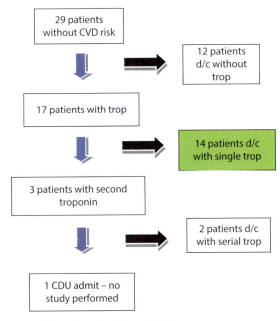

FIGURE 3-20. Clinical Chest Pain Audit *Low-Risk Group.*

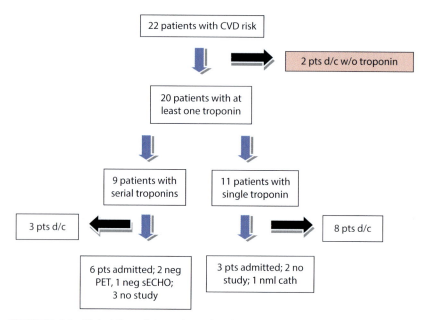

FIGURE 3-21. Clinical Chest Pain Audit *High-Risk due to CVD History.*

- Nine patients had two troponin levels; six were admitted; one patient had both troponin levels positive. Average time between troponin levels was 4.2 hours (1.5-14).
- Nine patients were admitted (three with one troponin; six with two troponin levels). Two of nine patients had positive troponin levels. Five of nine patients did not receive a study on admission; four patients received one single study; all studies were negative (stress ECHO [1], PET [2], card cath [1]).
- Two of 22 patients returned within 30 days. One patient presented with CV complaints (CHF). This patient was one of the prior nine admitted patients and one of the two patients with a positive troponin level.

High-Risk due to Abnormal ECG (Figure 3-22)
- Seven patients without CVD risk/history had abnormal ECGs.
- Four of seven patients had negative troponin levels and were discharged.
- Three patients did not have troponin levels and were discharged.
- There were no returns in 30 days.

Discussion
This was an introductory clinical audit on the EM practice at this site. The goal of these audits is to compare known literature or EBP with actual group practice, triggering introspection on the management of specific populations, and providing opportunity for practice adjustment.

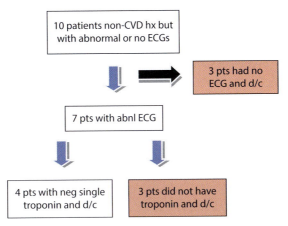

FIGURE 3-22. Clinical Chest Pain Audit *High-Risk due to Abnormal ECG.*

Low-Risk Group (Figure 3-20)

There is large variability of management of this specific population in this ED. The Marsan et al. article, based on the concept of reducing risk of CV events to <0.2%, suggests defining low-risk patients as those without CVD or risks, no cocaine usage, a nonischemic ECG, and a single negative troponin. Of the low-risk patients only 48% were managed with this approach. We identified three other management approaches to these low-risk patients: (1) discharge without a troponin level, (2) obtaining a second troponin level, and (3) admitting the patient to the CDU.

Notably all 29 patients had no 30-day returns and CV-associated evaluations. Certainly these data are limited to one facility review. Despite this, the outcomes are consistent with the pattern described in the Marsan et al. article.

It could be argued that three of these patients were overtested and overmanaged considering resource allocation and bed management. It could also be argued that the 14 patients discharged without a troponin level represent increased patient risk and should have had troponin levels assessed. The negative 30-day return record tempers this position. Is there a better approach?

High-Risk Group (Figures 3-21 and 3-22)

Of the higher risk group, not including the two patients with positive troponin levels who were admitted as inpatients, we identified five management approaches: (1) no troponin testing, (2) single troponin testing, (3) serial troponin testing, (4) admission to the CDU, (5) admission to an inpatient setting.

In observing the 30-day returns, the potentially higher risk group had predictable pattern of no returns *if the troponin level was negative during the prior visit.*

There were two patients potentially placed at risk as they were discharged without troponin levels.

Retrospectively, several patients had overtesting experiences. These patients had increased laboratory testing and extra procedures; all cardiology studies were negative.

If we admitted only those patients with first troponin positive this would reduce the admission rate from 16% to 3%, allowing open beds for potentially or proven more unstable or ill patients both in the CDU or inpatient. Would the rate of CV events, described by Marsan, be acceptable with this increased discharge rate?

Summary

Depending on stratification, we have identified up to nine variations of clinical practice for this low-risk population. Considering the literature on low-risk cardiovascular patients, some of the evaluation approaches observed may be more extensive than required for safely managing these patients.

Can you consider that our population has the potential to be similar in event pattern to the Marsan et al. study? Can we *apply* the other literature as surrogate? We in fact do this often in clinical practice. If you are in agreement that the populations are similar, are you willing to consider the risk potential as well?

Should we be testing as much? In this low-risk population? Should we be testing more? Are there specific patients that we can determine that require more or less testing?

Anthony Ferroggiaro

SEPSIS AUDIT

Based on the IHI Surviving Sepsis Campaign

Author's Comments

As per the introduction below, this audit is a direct comparison of a physician group's practice to Rivers et al. and the Surviving Sepsis Campaign goals. The study, a 6-month time period, identified 46 patients admitted with the ED diagnosis of sepsis. Thus these patients were identified within the ED evaluation and required the obligatory interventions.

Identifying these patients for the audit is fairly simple and can incorporate the ED patient log; the ICU patient log; and/or admission diagnosis and coding. The audit tool would be taken off the outstanding sepsis literature as well as the original Rivers' article.[41] Notably with this study, the average patient age was nearly exact to the Rivers' article; further supporting the concept that the local environment of practice can be similar and thus bound to the evidence-based literature. This is further affirmed with the doubling of mortality associated with a lack of ED resuscitation at the local site.

Politically this audit could be a nightmare; the data should be contained within the group and it may be necessary to have closed door meetings within the group. This is the reason for advocating a leveled audit summary depending on the audience: the auditor-physician needs to gain the group's attention to the data with an open, nondefensive attitude and thus the information must be limited to those outside of the group. This does not mean the knowledge and information can be ignored.

Leadership needs to own these results (if poor, and market them if good or improving) as sepsis management is increasingly on hospital quality dashboards and core measures. After acceptance of the current status of care and well-defined improvement plan needs to be initiated, ICU teams potentially aligned with ED teams, and champions anointed. There are several QI programs with national agencies that could be incorporated. (Please note that the database was not provided but the data are granular to physician identification).

Introduction

The Institute for Healthcare Improvement Surviving Sepsis Campaign has promoted a goal for hospitals: a 25% reduction in mortality from sepsis has the potential to save the lives of 200,000 people in the United States. Our hospital has adopted this sepsis focus and has committed to reduce sepsis mortality 25% by December 31, 20XX. The IHI program is developed from the Rivers et al. article, "Early Goal-Directed Therapy in the Treatment of Severe Sepsis and Septic Shock," *N Engl J Med.* 2001;345:1368-1377.

The Goals of the EGDT

IHI promotes the sepsis resuscitation bundle[†] (0-6 hours):

- Serum lactate measured
- Blood cultures obtained prior to antibiotic administration
- From the time of presentation, broad-spectrum antibiotics administered within 3 hours for ED admissions and 1 hour for non-ED ICU admissions
- In the event of hypotension and/or lactate >4 mmol/L (36 mg/dL): Deliver an initial minimum of 20 mL/kg of crystalloid (or colloid equivalent)
- Apply vasopressors for hypotension not responding to initial fluid resuscitation to maintain mean arterial pressure (MAP) >65 mm Hg
- In the event of persistent hypotension despite fluid resuscitation (septic shock) and/or lactate >4 mmol/L (36 mg/dL):
  - Achieve central venous pressure (CVP) of >8 mm Hg
  - Achieve central venous oxygen saturation ($ScvO_2$) of >70%

Demographics and General Description

This review includes 46 patients identified through ED logs and ICU logs who were admitted to the hospital in a 6-month period. Chart abstraction was standard: charts were collected via medical records and assessed with a simple audit tool developed using the IHI bundle elements. Of the 46 patients, 24 met the criteria for severe sepsis or septic shock, while 22 met the criteria for SIRS or sepsis. The mean patient age (68.4 ± 19.6 years old) was similar to the mean patient age in the Rivers' study (67.1 ± 17.4 years old).

[†]A "bundle" is a group of interventions related to a disease process that, when executed together, result in better outcomes than when implemented individually.

The mean LOS for all 46 patients in this study was 4.43 hours. These patients had an average ED LOS of >4 hours which is 74% the time allowed in the resuscitation bundle (0-6 hours). Though commendable that these patients can be quickly admitted, the ED has the opportunity to intervene with sepsis patients and initiate the bundle.

Early Identification
Early identification is needed in all sepsis patients. Protocols can be established within the triage system to assess for septic parameters. The median time of ED entry to first set of vital signs was 10 minutes, and 80% of the patients in this audit had vital signs within 20 minutes.

Time to MD evaluation was calculated in 35 patients, and had a median time of 8 minutes. Seventy-five percent of patients were seen within 36 minutes of the first set of vital signs. Ninety percent of the patients with MAP <65 were seen within 40 minutes of first vital signs. There is an inadequate delay between identification of the septic patient and the physician involvement. This process must be reviewed and the sequence of triage to notification of the physician must be reviewed.

Serum Lactate
Per IHI goal: *Given the high risk for septic shock, all patients with elevated lactate >4 mmol/L (36 mg/dL) will enter the early goal-directed therapy portion of the severe sepsis resuscitation bundle, regardless of blood pressure.* Only 9/46 patients (20%) had serum lactate assessment. More lactate screening is needed in these patients. More frequent requests by physicians will assist in increasing the awareness and successful sampling by the staff. A protocol-driven process will result in automatic sampling. Physicians need to review recommended responses to elevated lactate.

Blood Cultures Prior to Antibiotics
Per IHI Goal: *Thirty percent to 50% of patients presenting with a clinical syndrome of severe sepsis or shock have positive blood cultures. Therefore, blood should be obtained for culture in any critically ill septic patient. Collecting blood cultures prior to antibiotic administration offers the best hope of identifying the organism that caused severe sepsis in an individual patient.* Of the 46 patients within this audit, 43 (93.5%) patients had blood cultures obtained. Concerning within the process was an inadequate documentation of the timing and thus the sequence of obtaining blood cultures prior to antibiotics. Notably, other commentaries have advocated no delay with infusing antibiotics when blood cultures are delayed (poor venous access, etc). Further process improvement efforts can modify RN behavior for documentation of the high-frequency process.

Timely Antibiotics
Per IHI Goal: *From the time of presentation, broad-spectrum antibiotics administered within 3 hours for ED admissions and 1 hour for non-ED ICU admissions.* The mean time for receiving antibiotics within this audit was 3.09 hours with 65% of

the 46 patients receiving antibiotics within 3 hours. The maximum time for antibiotic infusion was 8.55 hours.

Over 30% of patients did not receive antibiotics prior to 3 hours. Most of the physicians and staff are unaware of this goal. Further education will heighten awareness with inclusion of protocols.

More concerning was that two patients received no antibiotics in the ED. One patient (#28) was diagnosed with pneumonia, had a 27% bandemia, was placed on dopamine, and had an ED LOS of 3.82 hours. A second patient (#43) had a diagnosis of unknown sepsis, ESRD, IDDM, and an ED LOS of 2.57 hours (Table 3-8).

Appropriate Antibiotics

Per IHI Goal: *Patients with severe sepsis or septic shock warrant broad-spectrum therapy until the causative organism and its antibiotic susceptibilities are defined.* In reviewing the data in Table 3-8, there is great variation on choice of antibiotics for patients with sepsis of unknown source. Most inadequate are patients receiving only a single agent. Further review of the broad-spectrum antibiotics revealed that only 42% of septic patients received two or more antibiotics in the ED (Figure 3-23).

Total IVF for Hypotension and/or Lactate >4

Per IHI Goal: *In the event of hypotension and/or lactate >4 mmol/L (36 mg/dL) deliver an initial minimum of 20 ml/kg of crystalloid (or colloid equivalent).* In the Rivers' EGDT subset comparing the isolated value of IV fluid resuscitation, the EGDT delivered 5 L resuscitation (to 3.5 L [p < .001]). The mean IVF volume

■ TABLE 3-8. Antibiotics for Unknown Source (N = 12)

Pt #	Antibiotic #1	Antibiotic #2
2	Ceftriaxone	
20	Levofloxacin	Imipenem
26	Zosyn	
28	None	
30	Zosyn	
31	Vancomycin	Zosyn
32	Vancomycin	Zosyn
35	Ampicillin	Gentamicin
36	Levofloxacin	
39	Levofloxacin	
43	None	
46	Imipenem	Vancomycin

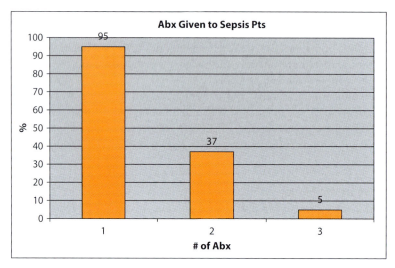

FIGURE 3-23. Percentage of septic patients receiving one or more antibiotics.

delivered to the patients with sepsis (MAP < 65) in this audit was 1.8 L (Table 3-9). Over 50% of patients did not receive the minimal entry IVF for resuscitation. Some patients received no IVF. Focusing on the IHI goal will increase the frequency of fluid administered. During the departmental presentation there were several questions regarding IVF resuscitation in the CHF patient (only 30% in this audit population). There is a difference between *pump failure* and *intravascular volume status* in which the latter could be low despite a dysfunctional pump. Resuscitation starts with adequate IVF; consideration of CVP monitoring to ensure adequate intravascular volume; consideration of vasopressors and dobutamine for cardiac support as necessary.

Vasopressors for Hypotension
Per IHI Goal: *Apply vasopressors for hypotension not responding to initial fluid resuscitation to maintain mean arterial pressure (MAP) ≥65 mm Hg. Only 37%*

■ TABLE 3-9. Relationship of Exit MAP, Age, IVF Resuscitation, Hospital LOS, and Mortality Rate		
Exit MAP	**≤65 mm Hg**	**>65 mm Hg**
Age	68.8 y	68.2 y
Tot IVF Mn/Md	1.82 L/1.10 L	1.19 L/ 1.00 L
LOS hospital (Mn)	**10.19 d**	8.07 d
Inhospital mortality	*31.3% (5/16)*	16.7% (5/30)

of patients with persistent hypotension had vasopressors initiated in the ED. Central venous access and aggressive vasopressor support if hypotension persists is required.

Maintain Adequate CVP

Per IHI Goal: *In the event of persistent hypotension despite fluid resuscitation (septic shock) and/or lactate >4 mmol/L (36 mg/dL) achieve central venous pressure (CVP) of ≥8 mm Hg.* For all patients, CVP was not obtained. Understandably this technique is often not part of the ED resuscitation in most sites due to the lack of equipment or a decision to expedite transfer. Concerning though is that lack of central venous access, only 3/46 patients (6.5%), but that 10 patients were placed on vasopressor support. This lack of procedure could be due to inadequate technique or inappropriate decision making. Ultrasound-guided CVC is the future and all the tools and training are present in the ED and group at this time. There is separate (increased) reimbursement for US-G CVC.

Disposition

There is no IHI goal with disposition. Of the 46 patients in this audit, 15 (37.5%) were placed in the ICU. Of the patients with persistent MAP <65 during the ED period, 9 (60%) were placed in the ICU. It is unclear why patients with persistent hypotension are placed on the general floor rather than in the ICU. This may be hospital flow pressure; if no ICU bed is available the septic patient resuscitation should be continued in the ED until the ICU is ready. Improvement work will involve increasing the collaboration between areas to potentially transfer some resources into the ED in the event of no ICU beds (ICU CCRNs, CVP monitoring, transition to intensivist management, etc).

Outcomes

In the Rivers et al. study, the treatment with EGDT resulted in an inhospital mortality of 30.5% compared to standard treatment 46.5% (p = 0.009). In comparison, even in this low patient volume audit, the pathophysiology of sepsis is evident (Table 3-9). Those patients with persistent ED hypotension fare worse than those with stable or stabilized BP. The inhospital mortality doubled and the hospital LOS increased 2 days when the patient exited the ED with MAP <65. What the ED does in the LOS of 4 hours makes a difference.

Critical Care Time

This is not an IHI goal. In all patients, 5.5% of the ED time was documented as critical care. Of the patients with entry MAP <65, 8% of the ED LOS was documented at critical care and this represents 22 minutes of critical care management in 4 hours.

This is P4P! No goal of critical care time can be advocated but all should agree that 5 minutes of each hour the septic patient is present in the ED is underdocumentation. All interventions can be billed separately; critical care time reimbursement increases with volume of time.

Summary

A more rigorous focus on the IHI Surviving Sepsis goals is necessary to ensure that adequate, comprehensive critical care treatment is provided for these patients within our ED. We need to increase early identification of the septic patient with a triage screening tool. The data presented support the need for a formal protocol much of which could be pre-physician evaluation activity. Physicians should be aware of the sepsis requirements as well as the changes (via literature review) in sepsis management and champion a high-quality protocol and ED management.

We need to increase lactate and ABG screening, blood cultures prior to antibiotics, earlier and more appropriate broad-spectrum antibiotics, infuse at least the minimum required intravenous fluids (20 cc/kg), provide more central access, and increase the use of ultrasound as a safer method of CVC placement. Once the CVC is placed we can aggressively support the blood pressure with vasopressors per the guidelines of persistent hypotension despite IV fluid resuscitation. We can dialogue with the ICU team to consider the indication for CVP assessment in the ED and absolutely we should be placing these patients in the ICU due to a higher need of intervention and the documented high mortality.

Next Steps

The Institute for Healthcare Improvement Surviving Sepsis Campaign has promoted a goal for hospitals: a 25% reduction in mortality from sepsis has the potential to save the lives of 200,000 people in the United States. Our hospital has adopted this sepsis focus and has committed to a goal of reducing sepsis mortality by 25% before December 31, 20xx.

In order to achieve this goal within our hospital, several steps can be promoted. The creation of collaborative clinical team within the ED and the ICU will clarify roles and activities per department. Further clarification from the team on the choices of antibiotics and vasopressors would standardize the care to these patients. Developing or incorporating a protocol for sepsis patients would be ideal that would support overall care, including a screening tool for triage and an order-set.

Ongoing education and feedback for the ED physicians are necessary once a guideline and standard has been affirmed. As per the audit, our patients have higher mortality with a reduced intervention, it will be necessary to change practice.

Anthony Ferroggiaro, MD

D-DIMER AND CT UTILIZATION AUDIT

Quality Committee

Author's Comments

Much of this study was prior to some EMRs incorporating the Wells score or PERC into documentation. It may be valuable to repeat this audit even with an EMR that has documentation for DVT and PE risk since use still varies even with increased awareness and opportunity for reminders via programming or forcing functions. Still, this audit has significant importance to patient safety and to overall departmental flow. The subsequent reduction of CT imaging using a pretest probability tool will reduce patient radiation exposure and will reduce patient throughput due to waiting for CT results.

Notable is that this audit was completed in a year between 2000 and 2010; the EM literature has had many affirming articles since this study. Crichlow and Venkatesh also showed incomplete use of pretesting (to mention only two).[42,43]

This was one of the first audits which incorporated some estimated costs. These amounts were simple calculations on the cost to the individual patients based on hospital billing. A more comprehensive number would be to include costs of valueless work such as radiologists reading unnecessary tests, ED RNs and lab techs completing unnecessary D-dimer processing. Taking the patient's perspective, it would be necessary to add lost hours in wages, etc. Please see the discussion on efficiency and opportunity cost in this section under The Operational Impact of Auditing.

Introduction

This study was undertaken to review the incidence of CT-positive PE findings within the ED evaluations, as well as to describe the physician practice pattern when considering PE has a potential diagnosis. There are multiple tests to assess pretest probability for PE; the most famous would be the Wells criteria (Table 3-10).

■ TABLE 3-10. Wells Criteria for Assessing Pretest Probability for PE

Criteria	Points
Suspected DVT	3.0
An alternative diagnosis consideration	3.0
Heart rate >100 bpm	1.5
Immobilization or surgery specifics	1.5
Previous DVT/PE	1.5
Hemoptysis	1.0
Malignancy specifics	1.0

Score Range	Mean Probability of PE	Interpretation of Risk
<2 points	3.6%	Low
2-6 points	20.5%	Moderate
>6 points	66.7%	High

Reprinted from Annals of Emergency Medicine. Vol. 63, Issue 4. "Clinical Policy: Critical Issues in the Evaluation and Management of Adult Patients Presenting to the Emergency Department With Seizure." pp 437-447. Copyright 2014, with permission from Elsevier.

The acknowledged clinical algorithm to managing the potential PE patients:

1. Assess the potential for PE in each patient
   a. Using a pretesting score such as the Wells criteria (clinical gestalt has been supported since this audit).[44]
2. Obtain the necessary evaluation based on the pretest score.
   a. Considering a low Wells score; the D-dimer assay could reliably exclude the PE diagnosis if the assay was negative.
   b. Considering a moderate to high Wells score; the D-dimer assay is not helpful in assessing potential for PE and should not be obtained; these patients should have an imaging evaluation.
      i. CT scanning for PE has been determined to be an acceptable EM practice considering alternatives such as pulmonary angiogram and V/Q nuclear scanning.

Methods

- The hospital HIS provided the initial database from laboratory services (D-dimer) and radiology services (CT angiogram for PE) which included ED site, patient name, MR#, date of service, D-dimer result if testing done, and CT chest for PE if completed.
- The time period was a single month—February 20XX.
- The clinical information was abstracted from EMR based on the EMR physician note. If no positive comment was documented according to specific Wells criteria components then that component was regarded as negative. Specifics of the data points with abstraction can be provided.
- Data were entered into the relational Microsoft Access database.
- Positive CT scans for PE were based on radiologist interpretation.
- D-dimer assay: Elevated (positive) results were >500 ng/mL FEU.

Results

General Distribution of Chief Complaint (Table 3-11)

Of the 383 patients assessed in this audit, 72% presented with CP and/or SOB as the chief complaint. Other complaints such as LE discomfort, swelling, syncope, or palpitations represented the remaining entry concerns.

■ **TABLE 3-11.** Distribution of Chief Complaint (Affirms Typical Presentation to Literature in This Local Population)

Number of Patients With CC	CC
181	CP
96	SOB
74	Other
14	LE complaints
12	Syncope
5	Palpitations

■ **TABLE 3-12.** Distribution of Chief Complaint With Subsequent Positive CT for PE (Affirms Typical Presentation to Literature in This Local Population)

Number of PE Patients With CC	CC
5	CP
5	SOB
2	Other
1	Syncope

Chief Complaint Associated With Positive CT for PE (Table 3-12)

Of the 13 CT-confirmed pulmonary emboli, patients complained of CP and/or SOB in 10/13 (77%).

Wells Score Distribution (Table 3-13)

Considering the Wells score distribution, less than 2 points represents low risk, 2-6 points represents moderate risk and >6 points represents high risk; 306 (80%) patients were assessed as low risk, 68 (18%) were moderate risk, and 8 (2%) were regarded as high risk.

Use Assessment
CT Usage (Table 3-13)

Of the 167 chest CT scans were completed to assess of PE, 13 (7.8%) were positive for PE. Interestingly, none of the patients with high probability Wells scores were found to have a PE. Eight patients were found with a PE and had moderate Wells risk while five patients with low Wells score were found with a PE.

D-Dimer Assay and CT Activity (Table 3-14)

Considering the promoted algorithm for assessing PE risk, patients with low Wells scores had D-dimer serum testing. Of the patients with elevated D-dimer levels (110/248), 49 had CT scanning for pulmonary embolus and three were confirmed positive for PE.

■ **TABLE 3-13.** Distribution of Patients According to Wells Score and CT Utilization/Result

Wells Score	#	Completed CT Scan	CT Scan + for PE	CT Scan – for PE
Low	306	119	5	114
Mod	68	46	8	38
High	8	3	0	3
Totals	383	167	13	154

> ■ **TABLE 3-14.** Relationship of Patients According to Wells Score, D-Dimer Result, and Completion of CT Scanning

Wells Score	D-Dimer Scale	# D-Dimer Tests	# CT Scans Completed	CT Scan + for PE
Low	>500 (+)	110	49	3
	<500 (−)	138	12	0
	Not done	58	58	2
Mod/high		48		

Of the patients with low D-dimer levels (138/248), 12 patients who had negative D-dimer testing received CT scans and none were identified as having a pulmonary embolus.

No D-dimer testing was obtained prior to 58 CT scans. Considering the frequency of negative D-dimer assay in the tested population was 56%, an estimated 32 of the 58 patients with no D-dimer testing would have negative D-dimer results. Considering the algorithm again, the potentially unnecessary CT scans would be 44 (12 + 32). This calculates to a rate of 37% unnecessary CT scans having low Wells criteria and negative D-dimer assay. Based on a $1200 charge for chest CT scans (conversation with radiology department) the calculated unnecessary costs for imaging outside of the Wells/PE algorithm would be $52,800.00 per month ($633,600.00 annually).

Considering the 76 patients with moderate to high probability on Wells score and the standard algorithm indicating that these patients should have CT imaging regardless of D-dimer level, 48 unnecessary D-dimer studies were performed. The calculated unnecessary costs for serum D-dimer testing would be $2688.00 per month ($32,256.00 annually).

Risk Assessment (Table 3-15)
Sixty-one patients with low Wells scores but elevated (positive) D-dimer assay results did not undergo CT scanning. Twenty-seven patients with moderate to high Wells scores did not receive CT scanning. The above activity is outside the recommended assessment algorithm and represents underassessment of potential PE patients. Considering the infrequency of angiogram or V/Q scanning within

> ■ **TABLE 3-15.** Relationship of Potentially Underevaluated Patients According to Wells Score, D-Dimer Result, and CT Scanning

Wells Score	#	No CT Completed	Had D-Dimer Testing	+ D-Dimer Result
Low	306	186	186	61
Mod	69	23		
High	8	5		

the ED these results do reflect an underevaluated population. This study did not determine those patients who were anticoagulated in the ED (treated for PE) and who did not receive full ED evaluation but may have subsequently obtained a study while admitted to the hospital.

Conclusion

There are well-recognized pretest probability tools developed through research that can assist the physician in evaluating the potential PE patient. Moreover, these tools when combined with the D-dimer assay result in a highly supportable negative predictive value for the determination of PE in each patient.

This study was undertaken to review the incidence of CT-positive PE findings within the ED evaluations, as well as to describe the physician practice pattern when considering PE as a potential diagnosis. Data were obtained on completed CT scans for PE and D-dimer studies for all EDs during February 20XX. Chart review abstracted elements of the Wells criteria to retrospectively determine the pretest probability for each patient who received CT scanning and D-dimer testing for PE.

Three-hundred eighty three patients were considered and assessed for PE. There were no instances of documentation of use of pretest assessment (Wells score number or other).

There is an underuse of pretest PE screening tools within the practice. This has resulted in a misuse of CT imaging and D-dimer testing on ED patients. Divisional practice should consider the potential risks of unnecessary or inadequate testing on ED LOS, patient satisfaction, cost to patients and insurers, risk of missed diagnosis and radiation exposure. Consideration of implementing education toward review of the Wells Criteria or other pretesting probability screens would be valuable. Divisional peer review monitoring of laboratory and imaging usage in this potential population would further reinforce the education and create a practice change.

Anthony Ferroggiaro

NSTEMI/CRUSADE FOCUSED REVIEW AND AUDIT

Quality Committee

Author's Comments

This is an important audit for most groups since STEMI core measures get the majority attention. Mechanistically, obtaining patients for this audit was enabled due to use of the laboratory database on troponin testing and identifying patients with + troponins as well as coding data for NSTEMI or USA. Incorporation of AHA guidelines allowed for outside reference and comparison and some matching patient demographics were used to affirm similar patient populations to the Crusade cohort.

One interesting finding in the audit was the identification of higher risk patients as those entering the ED with tachycardia. Physiologically this makes sense with associated troponin elevation on the second sample due to either demand ischemia or sympathetic response to ischemia. Opportunity for improvement was present with less than half the patients with NSTEMI receiving β-blockade.

Full Summary

The NSTEMI Focused Review and Audit was based on the CRUSADE National Quality Improvement Initiative (www.crusadeqi.com). *"CRUSADE is a national quality improvement initiative that is designed to increase the practice of evidence-based medicine for patients diagnosed with non-ST segment elevation acute coronary syndromes (NSTE ACS) (ie, unstable angina or NSTE myocardial infarction). The American College of Cardiology / American Heart Association Guidelines for the Management of Non-ST Segment Elevation Acute Coronary Syndromes are the "gold standard" by which appropriate care is defined."*

The NSTEMI Focused Review and Audit is a retrospective study using chart abstraction based on coding NSTEMI/Unstable Angina diagnoses; the patients reviewed have the discharge diagnosis of USA or NSTEMI.

The goals of this study were

1. To review our ED practice of NSTEMI care in comparison to national data
2. To review individual physician practice in regard to NSTEMI care
3. To assess the level of ED involvement with cardiology in NSTEMI care
4. To compare initial cardiology treatment with hospitalist treatment of NSTEMI patients

General Data and History

Seventy-four charts were reviewed between sites. Forty-seven physicians were included in the study.

Demographics (Table 3-16)

In comparison with the CRUSADE national data, 38% of the Focused Review patients were female (CRUSADE 40%), with an average age of 71 years (CRUSADE 67 ± 14 years). According to Cardiovascular Past Medical History, the review had similar frequencies of DM, prior cath/PCI, and prior CABG. It could be concluded that the Focused Review population (our local population) represented the CRUSADE population.

Time to ECG for NSTEMI Patients (Table 3-16)

In comparison to the goal of less than 9 minutes for STEMI patients (usually presenting with CP), the NSTEMI patient ECG averages at all sites but two were increased. This may be due to the varied presentation of this population, including dyspnea and weakness as clinical mimics of chest pain.

Evaluation (Table 3-17)

Again in comparison to the CRUSADE national data, there was similar frequencies in the NSTEMI population of presentation with tachycardia, hypotension and in congestive heart failure.

Diagnosis of NSTEMI (Table 3-17)

Seventy-six percent of patients received the diagnosis of NSTEMI from an elevated cardiac enzyme pattern, whereas 18 patients (of 74) remained without enzyme

■ **TABLE 3-16.** General Data and History

Hospital	No. Patients	No. MDs	M	F	Mean Age (Years)	# DM	# Prior MI	#Prior PCI	# Prior CABG	# Charts With Time of Eval*	Average T to ECG (ECG T – Entry T)	Average Time to Eval (Eval T – Entry T)
	15	11	10	5	67	6	2	5	1	16	8.8 (18)	9.9
	19	10	15	4	71	7	3	6	3		9.1 (19)	
	10	8	6	4	70	6	5	1	2		14.8 (13)	
	18	10	8	10	80	6	4	2	3		38 (18)	
	12	8	7	5	67	5	1	4	1		24 (12)	
Totals	**74**	**47**	**46**	**28**	**71**	**30**	**15**	**18**	**10**			
%					38%	39%	17%	25%	14%			
CRUSADE					40%	67 ± 14	33%	30%	21%	19%		

* Evaluation Times and ECG Times included those patients excluded from subsequent NSTEMI Evaluation.

■ **TABLE 3-17.** Evaluation Description

Hospital	No. Patients	Mean Age (Years)	# HR >100 in ED	# SBP <95 in ED	# in CHF in ED	Final # w/ + enzymes	Final # With All Neg	# Dx With NSTEMI in ED	ED: # w/ + enzymes	ED: # ECG + STD/Trop Neg	# Dx on Inpt Trop
	15	67	5	0	5	10	5	7	5	2	3
	19	71	2	1	3	13	6	10	6	4	3
	10	70	3	0	4	7	3	6	4	2	3
	18	80	5	3	1	15	3	9	7	2	6
	12	67	4	0	3	11	1	3	2	1	8
Totals	74	71	19	4	16	56	18	35	24	11	23
%			26%	5%	22%	76%		63%	69% (24/35)	31%	
CRUSADE			23%	4%	24%	92%				31%	

elevation throughout hospitalization. Of the 56 patients with elevated cardiac enzymes, 63% were diagnosed with NSTEMI/USA in the emergency department, with 69% showing elevated enzymes with the emergency department laboratory values. Eleven patients (31% of NSTEMI ED patients) were diagnosed with NSTEMI/USA based on ECG changes, consistent with the CRUSADE average also of 31%.

Management in the ED—Troponin or ECG-Positive Patients (Table 3-18)

Thirty-five patients were diagnosed with NSTEMI in the ED. Accordingly, CRUSADE advocates initiating medical therapy on these patients within the first 24 hours. As is evident from the following chart, the frequency of medication initiated in the ED was lower than the CRUSADE 24-hour frequencies. It is difficult to consider this comparison and make critical interpretations as the ED usually represents the first 3 hours of acute MI care for these patients and that there is limited evidence-based literature defining the benefit of ED management. The range of ED medical intervention is ongoing in the literature, and there appears no consensus upon which to base practice. Nevertheless, as the diagnosis of NSTEMI was completed in the ED, medical intervention may be pursued. Of note, 57% of NSTEMI patients received cardiology consultation (phone or bedside evaluation) while in the ED. Those patients who received ED cardiology consultation had more medical intervention (subreview), but outcomes are limited due to patient numbers. Twenty-six percent ED NSTEMI patients were admitted to a cardiologist.

Management in the ED—Troponin or ECG-Negative Patients, Subsequent Second Troponin Positive vs Negative

Twenty-one patients presented to the ED with ischemic symptoms, nonspecific ECG findings and a nonelevated cardiac enzyme test had elevated cardiac enzymes with the second enzyme sample as inpatients. In comparison to the ED NSTEMI patients, these patients received aspirin as frequently, but all other medical intervention was minimally provided. In comparing the patients who remained without elevation in cardiac enzymes throughout the hospitalization, a similar frequency of treatment was provided. In conclusion, without elevation in enzymes or diagnostic ECG, the ED MD will have difficulty determining which patients will subsequently infarct. A subgroup analysis of these two populations was completed, based on the risk stratification described in the article, "Practical Implementation of the Guidelines for Unstable Angina/Non-ST-Segment Elevation Myocardial Infarction in the Emergency Department"[45] (Table 3-19). It appears that increased age and on presentation any abnormal ECG may increase the likelihood that the patient will have an infarction. Therapy in both groups could be further focused based on risk stratification.

Procedures/β-Blockade Subanalysis

Referring to the ED presentation (Chapter 2), a total of 19 patients presented to the ED with tachycardia. Of those 19 patients with ischemic symptoms and heart rates >100 beats per minute, 42% received β-blockade (BB contraindicated patients

■ **TABLE 3-18.** Management of ED Troponin-Positive or ECG-Positive Patients

Hospital	No. Patients ED Pos	# Given ASA	In ED, # Given BB	BB Contra	In ED, # Given Heparin	In ED, # Given GP2B3A I	In ED, # Given Clopidogrel	In ED, # Given NTG	# Pts + ED Trop w/ CV Consult	# Pts + ED NSTEMI – CV Admit
	7	6	1	2	5	4	1	6	6	3
	10	8	3	2	4	2	0	6	3	3
	6	3	2	2	2	1	1	3	5	2
	9	5	2	1	2	0	0	3	5	1
	3	2	1	0	0	0	0	2	1	0
Totals	35	24	9	7	13	7	2	20	20	9
%		69%	32%		37%	20%	6%	57%	57%	26%
CRUSADE		96%	90%		82%	47%	54%			

■ TABLE 3-19. Relationship of NSTEMI Patients to Non-NSTEMI Patients Based on Entrance Factors

	ED Trop and ECG Neg; Subsequent Second Trop Pos (N = 20)	All Negative—ED and Admission (N = 18)
Average age	73	67
[% Age >70]	[65%]	[50%]
(% Age <60)	(10%)	(33%)
DM	35%	33%
Normal ECG	10%	44%

excluded). Of those patients presenting with tachycardia, 16 (84%) had ED troponin elevation or second set enzyme elevation while hospitalized. These data are concerning. As the ED has the role in stabilization and perhaps early intervention in a presumed infarcting patient; some opportunities are more clinically clear and less risk prone from medical intervention aspect. β-Blockade in the clinically ischemic, tachycardic patient should be advocated.

In considering risk assessment in the ED, the PURSUIT trial[46] contained a review of clinical features and the increased incidence of M & M. Heart rate was second only to age in significance as a predictor of poor outcome.

Conclusions
This Focused Review assisted in defining the ED NSTEMI population as well as describing the level of medical intervention provided to these patients.

Recommendations can be provided according to the subgroups, and these are defined in the initial summary above.

Recommendations
ED Troponin-Positive or ECG-Positive Patients
Aggressive medical intervention should be provided in the ED for patients with the diagnosis of NSTEMI, either ED troponin-positive or diagnostic ECG. Focus should be on antiplatelet therapies; β-blockade should also be provided.

1. Increase cardiology consultation in the ED and request cardiology to admit all patients with myocardial infarction or ECG-positive findings.
2. Increase use of aspirin (162-325 mg).
3. Increase use of β-blockers.
   a. Relative contraindications to β-blockers (taken from AHA STEMI 2004 recommendations):
      i. Recent cocaine use
      ii. HR <60

    iii. SBP <100

    iv. Mod-severe LV failure

    v. Shock

    vi. Second- to third-degree AVB

    vii. RAD

b. Significant are the data on BB usage and tachycardia in this review:

    i. Aggressive use of BB in the population should be advocated.

       1. In our study, 84% of patients with HR >100 on ED presentation had positive troponins.

    ii. In considering risk assessment in the ED, the PURSUIT[46] trial contained a review of clinical features and the increased incidence of morbidity and mortality. Heart rate was second only to age in significance as a predictor of poor outcome.

4. Increase use of heparin agents. LMWH is preferable to UFH and has been found to be as effective for NSTEMI patients—SYNERGY,[47] ESSENCE,[48] TIMI IIB.[49] Moreover, LMWH have advantages of less monitoring and fewer medication-related side effects. Adjust LMWH dosage with renal insufficiency.

5. Consider use of clopidogrel (300 mg) with or prior to cardiology consultation—CURE.[50]

6. Consider use of GPI with cardiology consultation.

ED Troponin and ECG Negative

In reflection of the Fesmire article,[51] the ED MD may be required to balance a projected specific benefit from the acute medical intervention of ACS in the ED (despite no current rigorous ED-oriented evidence-based guidance) with a conservative practice. It appears difficult to define with certainty the higher risk population. Thus the QC could provide these recommendations to MDs:

1. Use of current guidelines for stratification of CP patients to identify an ED troponin-negative, high-risk population. See Table 1: "Practical Implementation of the Guidelines for Unstable Angina/Non-ST-Segment Elevation Myocardial Infarction in the Emergency Department."[45]

    a. Consistent with the above article, a subgroup analysis within this study revealed both increased age and an abnormal ED ECG may support increased risk of infarction.

2. Timely ED cardiology consultation must occur with the higher risk population.

3. Consideration of more aggressive medical management in the above population with or without cardiology involvement.

    i. The agents BB, clopidogrel, heparin, and GPI have varied safety profiles that may allow increased frequency or opportunity for use.

Anthony Ferroggiaro, MD

DOUBLE AUDIT OF NEONATAL SEPSIS PRACTICE COMPLIANCE

Guideline for Fever in the Less Than 60-Day Old

Author's Comments

This audit affirms the value of sequential clinical auditing as a performance improvement method. The summary is a combination of two exact audits with 1 year time period between and salutes group awareness as well as other interventions.

As mentioned in the introduction, single peer review cases can trigger a clinical audit as in this case. Several cases of incomplete evaluations were identified by the pediatric hospitalist group and were referred for review. The first audit confirmed gaps in evaluation. A standard was then created with the pediatric medical leadership and promoted throughout the associated EDs. Interventions are described within the summary.

Also noted was an operational issue within the ordering of urine cultures that once addressed resulted in ease of completion and higher compliance.

A recent Pediatrics article[52] affirms the variation of clinical management of this pediatric population evident in this audit.

Introduction

This is the completion of a quality audit on the compliance of clinical evaluation defined as standard of practice within the Clinical Practice Guideline for Pediatric Fever of Unknown Source in Infants <60 Days Old. The initial evaluation included 119 cases of patients less than 60 days old and seen in one of six EDs. The date range was from August 24, 20XX, through August 24, 20XX. A summary of this report was provided to all physicians as well as to the Medical Directors and Board (above).

Methods

The follow-up audit was completed and included exact methodology to the first audit. The date range for patient selection was August 24, 20XX-20XX.

The second audit contained 99 patients; the first audit contained 119 patients. The EMR query narrowed the field of patients using the chief complaint of "fever" and under "age": "<60 days." Patients older than 61 days old were excluded.

Fever was defined within this study per the guideline and had to be a numeric entry into the EMR. The physician could either record the ED temperature or record the reported fever value from the parental history. Twelve cases of unrecorded temperature in the EMR were left to the reviewer's interpretation based on the subsequent evaluative actions by the ED MD. If the MD initiated an evaluation, blood or urine, or more, etc, then this was interpreted as evidence of "fever" and concern for sepsis. Likewise, if the physician did not note a temperature and did not evaluate for sepsis the case would be given a nonfebrile status.

FUS was designated if no symptoms or signs by history or on examination allowed a diagnosis. If the physician noted a possible source (cellulitis, URI symptoms, and gastroenteritis symptoms), then this would be noted and the case excluded from FUS review. Required URI symptoms are both cough and rhinorrhea to meet the inclusion; vomiting and diarrhea would meet the gastroenteritis inclusion.

Data on the evaluation (imaging; blood and urine evaluations; and procedures) and results were obtained through EMR review, including microbiology data.

Outcome and disposition data were obtained through electronic discharge summaries for all admitted patients and/or EMR review. Subsequent return data were based on whether the patient reentered the system within a week after the initial evaluation.

Results
Prevalence of Bacteremia
The prevalence of bacteremia in the first audit (Table 3-20) was consistent with epidemiological patterns in the literature; the younger the patient the higher the likelihood of bacteremia. Of neonates determined to have FUS, 3/31 (9.7%) had bacteremia in the less than 30-day-old group whereas 1/27 (3.7%) had bacteremia in the 31- to 60-day-old group. These data confirmed the consistency of the audit sample as representative of national patterns and affirmed transposing the management advocacy in the EB literature and guidelines to the local practice.

Overall, in the less than 30-day olds, including both FUS and fever with source, specific bacteremia results included one patient with GABHS bacteremia in cellulitis presentation, one patient with GNR bacteremia in UTI, one patient with E coli bacteremia in UTI, and one patient with GBS bacteremia in a treated UTI. In the 31- to 60-day olds, specific bacteremia results included one patient with GBS bacteremia in GBS + mother (34 day old).

Evaluation of 1-30 Day Olds (Table 3-21)
In reviewing the FUS evaluation for this age group, compliance with the guideline recommended workup (CBC + Urine + BC + LP + Admission [full evaluation]) went from 68% (15/24) to 96%. In the first audit, 92% (22/24) of the FUS patients were admitted and this increased as well to 96%. Those patients receiving the recommended antibiotics also increased from 81% (18/22) to 92%.

Evaluation of 31-60 Day Olds (Table 3-22)
In reviewing the FUS evaluation for this age group in the first audit, 10/18 patients (56%) had evaluations c/w guideline. This increased to 92% after intervention.

The admission rate in this population increased from 17% to 80%.

Appropriate ED antibiotic treatment rate increased from 61% to 85%.

■ TABLE 3-20. Prevalence of Bacteremia in First Audit		
	Age ≤30 days old	Age ≥31 days old
All patients (5/119)	8.5% (4/47)	1.4% (1/72)
In FUS patients (4/58)	9.7% (3/31)	3.7% (1/27)

■ **TABLE 3-21.** Summary of Two Audits—1 to 30-Day-Old Patients

Population	Focus	Audit 1	Audit 2 Postintervention	Comments
1-30 d		24/36	26/37	Included documented fever population (20 patients) and no fever population (6 patients) who had septic workup
	Compliance with workup	68% (15/24)	96% (25/26)	Exclusions: (1) Patient with spinal bifida, sp surg, no LP; (2) family refused LP and admission, no 7 d return; (3) family refused admission, no 7 d return. One patient without fever, but full septic workup was discharged
	Admission rate	92% (22/24)	96% (23/24)	See above
	ED Antibiotics	81% (18/22)	92% (22/24)	
				Note: 11 patients without fever and without ED septic workup who were discharged from the ED; no returns in 7 d

Discussion

This was a completion of the Neonatal Sepsis Audit initiated in August 20XX. The format was straightforward, a comparison of current practice based on the advocacy of a pediatric practice guideline. The implications of this audit and the effort to improve the clinical practice of this specific population are clear based on historical practice patterns and risk management issues.

After the first audit (data present in Tables 3-23 and 3-24), in relation to the data, the following recommendations were forwarded:

Conclusions and Recommendations from Audit 1

1. The evaluations for these specific patients varied per site and per physician.
   a. In general, there is lack of compliance with the guideline recommendations in both the under-30-day population and the 31- to 60-day population. The significant risk of morbidity and mortality associated with this presentation requires 100% compliance with the guideline evaluation.

■ **TABLE 3-22.** —Summary of Two Audits—31- to 60-Day-Old Patients

Population	Focus	Audit 1	Audit 2 Postintervention	Comments
31-60 d		18/60	25/62	
	Compliance with workup	56% (10/18)	92% (23/25)	One patient had absent urine evaluation; one patient discharged from the ED had hx of maternal GBS+ and did not meet low-risk SBI criterion
	Admission rate	17% (3/18)	80% (20/25)	Five patients were discharged; 1/5 did not meet compliance as above
	ED Antibiotics	61% (11/18)	85% (17/20)	
				Note: Five patients were discharged; no returns in 7 d
				Note: 13 patients had no fever but received septic workup; 11/13 met compliance with guideline; one return within 7 d

b. Specific physicians at each site were exceptional in their care while other physicians did not meet the standard of care.

   i. Physicians and sites should review and discuss the Pediatric Fever Guidelines to ensure knowledge of the standard of care.

   ii. Physicians should change practice in accordance with the guidelines.

     1. In the 1- to 30-day population: Specific concern on the performance of the LP in this population should be addressed.

       a. Recommendations would include: Pediatric CME; observation at children's hospital site with a pediatric emergency medicine specialist; internal procedure lab.

     2. In the 31- to 60-day population: Understanding of SBI criteria and use of such criteria in combination with direct discussion with PCP (and thus close follow-up) is the standard of care. Physicians should not avoid LP in this population if SBI criteria not met.

     3. Antibiotic appropriate for age should be discussed. There was wide variance in approach in the 1- to 30-day sample with more consistency in the older sample.

■ **TABLE 3-23.** First Audit Data—Less Than 30-Day-Old Patients

Site	MD Name	MR #	Age in Days	Urine	WBC	Blood Cx	LP	Admit Y/N	Abx	Outcome
			17	True	True	True	True	True	+	UTI/S Ro; Neg BC
			12	True	True	True	True	True	+	Neg Cx
			18	True	True	True	True	True	A, Cefo	Neg Cx
			20	True	True	True	True	True	A, Cefo	Neg Cx
			26	True	True	True	True	True	A, Cefo	Neg Cx
			24	True	True	True	True	True	A, Ro	viral syn
			11	True	True	True	True	True	A, Ro	UTI/S Ro; Neg BC
			23	True	True	True	True	True	A, Cefo	Neg Cx
			23	True	True	True	True	True	A, Cefo	UTI/S Ro; BC+
			25	True	True	True	True	True	A, Cefo	Viral mening
			11	True	True	True	True	True	A, Cefo	Neg Cx
			7	True	True	True	True	True	A, G	Neg Cx
			22	True	True	True	True	True	A, G, Acy	UTI/S Ro; BC neg
			4	True	True	True	True	True	N	Neg Cx
			24	True	True	True	True	True	U	Neg Cx
			7	True	True	True	False	True	Cefo	UTI/S Ro/BC neg
			3	True	True	True	False	True	N	Neg Cx
			22	True	True	True	False	True	Ro	UTI/S Ro; BC pos E coli
			11	True	True	False	True	True	A, Cefo	Viral Syn
			25	True	False	False	False	True	N	Neg Cx
			28	False	True	True	True	True	Ro	GNB BACT/ UCX NEG
			30	False	False	False	True	True	Ro	Neg Cx
			11	False	False	False	False	False	N	na
			25	False	False	False	False	False	N	na

2. There is a culture-ordering failure at several sites.

   a. Laboratory should automatically perform urine culture based on age of presentation (pediatric patients) without the formal request (ie, the EMR ordering of the urine culture).

   b. Rare failures of blood culture ordering need to be reviewed operationally.

TABLE 3-24. First Audit Data—31- to 60-Day-Old Patients

Site	MD	MR #	Age	Urine	WBC	Blood Cx	LP	Hx= Low Risk for SBI	Discussion With PCP	Abx	Admit Y/N	Outcome	Returns
			42	True	True	True	True	True	True	Ro	False	Neg Cx	Y
			31	True	True	True	True	True	True	Ro	False	Neg Cx	N
			57	True	True	True	True	True	True	Ro	False	Neg Cx	Y
			36	True	True	True	True	True	True	Ro	False	Neg Cx	N
			51	True	True	True	True	False	True	Ro	False	Neg Cx	na
			34	True	True	True	True	False	False	A, Cefo	True	BC=GBBHS	na
			37	True	True	True	True	False	False	Ro	True	Neg Cx	na
			44	True	True	True	False	True	True	na	False	Neg Cx	N
			48	True	True	True	False	True	True	Ro	False	UTI/S Ro; Neg BC	N
			48	True	True	True	False	True	True	Ro	False	Neg Cx	N
			34	True	True	True	False	True	False	N	False	Neg Cx	N
			39	True	True	True	False	False	True	N	False	Neg Cx	N
			33	True	True	True	False	False	True	Ro	False	UTI/S Ro; Neg BC	N
			37	True	True	True	False	False	False	N	True	Neg Cx	na
			55	True	True	False	False	True	True	Ro	False	UTI/S Ro - No BC	N
			42	False	False	False	False	True	False	N	False	na	N
			53	False	False	False	False	True	False	N	False	na	N
			53	False	False	False	False	False	True	N	False	Neg Cx	Y

3. Extra-ED behavior must be addressed.
   a. PCPs and admitting staff may not be supportive of the standards. During chart review, there were frequent references to PCP decision making via phone on the management of the ED patient. Some ED physicians appeared reliant on this "consultation" to support the incompleteness of examination. The reliance of the ED MD on the above physicians to counter the necessity for full sepsis workup has weak medical legal defense in comparison to completing the evaluation.
      i. The Pediatric Fever Guideline should be provided to all involved in the care of this population in order to define and support the ED role in evaluation. There may be a lack of knowledge of the standard of care in the community.
   b. The reliance of the ED MD on the above physicians to counter the necessity for full sepsis workup has weak medical legal defense in comparison to completing the evaluation.
      1. This statement must be discussed at all site meetings during the guideline and data review.
      2. An approach may be recommended to address distinct cases in which the inability to complete the evaluation, not inappropriate decision making, causes delay in care and challenges compliance.
         a. On example of this is the inability to obtain CSF. An approach algorithm may be suggested/discussed at each site. Most sites/physicians may have similar approach that could be universal.
            i. Primary ED MD attempt twice
            ii. Second ED MD attempt
            iii. Discussion with admitting MD on decision to hold antibiotics prior to third LP attempt (by admitting MD).
               1. Discussion must be documented.
               2. Consideration of imaging assistance.

After the first audit, in consideration of the recommendations, several interventions to improve care were initiated prior to the second audit:

- November 20XX: Publication of the audit summary and guideline to all physicians
- December 20XX: Division Grand Rounds presentation
- December 20XX: Quality Committee presentation and strategic planning on focused divisional education. Subsequent committee physician members advocated for focus on the guideline as well as discussed the audit data at the respective division meetings and with divisional members.
- January 20XX: Contacted 12 physicians identified through the audit with care outside the guideline recommendations. Discussion of the cases via phone or

e-mail or both, including letter of introduction, the specific case summary, and a copy of the guideline for review.

- February 20XX: Presentation of the audit and findings to X division.
- Fall 20XX: Presentation of the audit and findings to Y division.

Interventions were very specific and largely educational. Two notable exceptions were first, with the initial audit, identification of operational conflict (confusion) over ordering pediatric urine evaluations resulting in missing cultures. The answer was to combine the two tests into a single order. Secondly, via a request to the Simulation Lab, a Laerdal neonatal LP simulation tool was purchased to encourage LP practice at all sites. Unfortunately this tool did not become available until midsecond audit and thus played no role in the outcomes. Advocacy of simulation, including the introduction and use of this LP tool, is advancing in EM and will provide future focus.

In conclusion, there is a dramatic and significant change in practice observed through the data. Remarkable is the physician modification of practice largely based on observation of group and individual patterns of practice and personal communication of specific cases in relation to the standard of practice. This change is the result of many factors: the singular introspection by individual physicians, the appropriate interventional quality improvement tactics and emphasis, the validity of guidelines developed from evidence-based medicine, and the attitude or willingness of an organization, and again its individuals, to adjust practice for the betterment of the patient.

Addendum

According to the Clinical Practice Guideline for Pediatric Fever of Unknown Source (FUS) in Infants <60 Days Old, there are several basic evidence-based rules.

Rule "A": Laboratory Evaluation: Every infant <60 days with FUS should have the following five laboratory tests:

CBC with diff, BC, UA, UrineCx, LP with CSF analysis and Cx.

CXR is optional but advocated with respiratory symptoms.

(Exception: infants 31-60 days of age meeting criteria for "low risk for SBI," above and available reliable caretakers and follow-up and PCP agrees with plan of care and antibiotics will not be started, need NOT necessarily have LP done)

Rule "B": All infants with FUS under 31 days of age should be admitted to the hospital.

Rule "C": Infants between 31 and 60 days who meet "low risk for SBI" criteria, above, and have negative results on all lab tests, above, with *reliable caretakers* and *close, reliable follow-up* may be managed as outpatients. *This disposition, with or without parenteral ceftriaxone prior to discharge, should be made only if all appropriate lab studies have been obtained.* Infants who do not meet "low risk for SBI" criteria and/or have one or more positive lab tests should be admitted to hospital.

Anthony Ferroggiaro, MD

ABDOMINAL PAIN, UNCLEAR ETIOLOGY, AUDIT

Quality Committee

Author's comments

Abdominal pain is a frequent presentation to the ED. Several high-risk presentations are associated with abdominal pain and monitoring the practice pattern of abdominal pain evaluation would have operational value considering the use of CT imaging and overall LOS. Technically and politically, it is invaluable to affirm good care—as in the higher risk population in this audit who received more comprehensive evaluations and more advocacy of returning to the ED if worsening.

Another aspect of combining other departmental or hospital goals within the clinical audit is the evaluation of pain control within the abdominal pain population. Indeed, since hospitals are focused on HCAHPS (Hospital Consumer Assessment of Healthcare Providers and Systems) survey and VBP, combining this measure into any audit will provide increased opportunity for practice reflection.

Note: Guaiac examinations were advocated within a limited population during the time of this audit; more literature has since reduced the indications for stool heme sampling as well as rectal examinations. This exposed the value of clinical auditing; as science discovers, the literature that directs patient care changes and the subsequent clinical audits should reflect those changes expected in practice. Importantly, the group of physicians being audited should be aware of these changes either through individual efforts or group learning and interaction. Clinical auditing can drive knowledge translation.

Included is a sample data form for abstraction.

Background

This is a report on the Quality Committee study of the group's practice in the evaluation and management of patients with abdominal pain of unclear etiology. Prior to this Quality Committee review, there has been no formal study on patient care on the presentation of undifferentiated abdominal pain. As abdominal pain of unclear etiology (APUE) is both "high risk," multiple etiologies could lead to increased morbidity and mortality, and "high volume," 5% to 10% of ED visits are abdominal pain related; it is a focus for quality of care review. The goals of this review were (1) to understand our patient population in comparison with national policy and population, (2) to examine the MD's approach to evaluation and management of the APUE patient, (3) to identify risk-prone activities defined either by literature/policy or by consensus, and (4) to reinforce areas of high-quality practice.

There are two subreviews within this evaluation. The first was to observe use of the EMR as a data tool. The method was to review how frequently the ED physician was documenting time of start and finish of evaluation. The goal was to encourage documentation such that length of service (LOSe) could be divided from length of stay (LOS). It is considered that the LOSe, or physician activity, is not the driver of increased LOS, but there are no local data to support this impression. The second subreview was to assess pain management activity by physicians including the frequency and timeliness of pain medication, and to reinforce patient satisfaction goals with pain management in the ED.

The structure of the review was based on the sections of the ACEP Clinical Policy "Critical Issues for the Initial Evaluation and Management of Patients Presenting With a Chief Complaint of Nontraumatic Acute Abdominal Pain,"[53] which was forwarded via e-mail to all physicians. Charts were identified using the coding for "abdominal pain of unclear etiology."

Final Summary and Recommendations for Clinicians

- Increase EMR documentation of starting time and completion time of service (see below—Section One).

- Increase recommendation for reevaluation in <2 days, especially in all high-risk patients (age >55 years and/or with vascular or immunocompromising diseases). It is advocated that these patients should return to the ED, considering the high frequency of admission, risk of pathology, and accessibility to further imaging studies, testing, and consultation (Sections One and Three).

- Increase frequency of gynecological and guaiac examinations (Section Two). There is minimal time expenditure for completion of guaiac evaluation and value is added to the evaluation. Gynecological examinations may decrease the frequency or need and/or improve the accuracy of subsequent imaging.

- Increase frequency of serial examinations.

- Maintain and/or increase the comprehensive examinations in all high-risk patients (Section Three).

- Increase frequency of consideration (documentation) of appendicitis (Section Four).

- Increase frequency of pregnancy testing due to the possibility of ectopic pregnancy in the APUE patient and due to the uncertainty of pregnancy/fetal effects with medicinal or radiation exposure (Section Four).

- Increase frequency of cardiac evaluation in high-risk patients with APUE (Section Four).

- Emphasis on earlier pain medication administration. Consider pain treatment prior to completing full examination to improve patient satisfaction and to improve the clinical evaluation.

Section One: Diagnosing Undifferentiated Abdominal Pain (Table 3-25)

One hundred thirty-five charts were reviewed. Fifty four physicians were reviewed.

Length of Service: Forty-nine percent of EMRs had both start time and discharge time recorded. Further review of the 66 charts will assist in comparison of LOSe to LOS.

General Data: Roughly 80% of charts had APUE as the primary diagnosis; 29 cases with APUC or APEU as secondary; example: vomiting as primary. Follow-up recommendations varied in length of time; the ACEP Clinical Policy advocates

■ TABLE 3-25. Diagnosing Undifferentiated Abdominal Pain

Hospital	No. Patients	No. MDs represented	M	F	% Charts Docu Length of Eval[a]	% Pts Given Dx AP, Unk Cause	% Pts Given Follow-up <2 days	No. Pts Returned to ED	No. Pts Admitted on Return to ED	No. Pts With Identified Dx on Return	No. Pts With Dx Common Missed Dx[b]
	29	13	14	15	7/29	29/29	14/29	7	1	4/7	0
	31	13	14	17	22/31	23/31	13/31	6	0	0	0
	36	13	10	26	30/36	22/36	19/36	5	1	0	0
	39	15	13	26	7/39	32/39	10/39	8	3	5/8	0
na	135	54	51	84	66/135	106/135	56/135	18/135	5	9/16	0
					49%	79%	41%	13%	(5/18) 28%		
									(5/135) 4%		

[a]Length of eval = T charts documenting both start of eval time and discharge time.
[b]AAA, appy, EP, MI, diverticulitis, perf viscus, mesenteric ischemia, bowel obstruction.

"timely follow-up." Consensus in the Quality Committee advocates <2 days as a recommendation. It is unclear by this study how feasible this time period is for patients. Secondary recommendations on discharge could be to return to the ED for reevaluation if no improvement or worsening in <2 days.

A small number of patients returned to the ED, and over one-quarter were admitted. Though none of these patients had "common missed diagnoses," evaluations on second visits clarified the etiology of the abdominal pain in over 50% of patients. This is supportive of the recommendations by the ED physicians to return to the ED if no improvement or worsening pain, and is an excellent support of risk management and quality practice behavior.

Recommendations
- Increase EMR documentation of start and completion of service.
- Increase disposition with the direction for reevaluation in <2 days.
- Encourage to return to the ED if no improvement or worsening.

Section Two: Evaluating Abdominal Pain (Table 3-26)
General Data: Both guaiac evaluation and the gynecological evaluation were infrequently part of the examination of patients presenting with APUE. The ACEP Clinical Policy provides no direction on the indications for both of these examinations. The Quality Committee would advocate the value of both examinations for comprehensive evaluations. There is minimal time expenditure for completion of guaiac evaluation and value is added to the evaluation. Gynecological examinations may decrease the frequency or need and/or improve the accuracy of subsequent imaging. It is recognized, and will be addressed, that there are significant barriers within the ED for the timely completion of the gynecological examination. Future efforts will be to strengthen the RN and staffing expectation of the gynecological examination in AP patients.

	No. Patients	% Pts With Pelvic or Bimanual	% Pts With Guaiac	% Pts With Documented Reevals (Serial Exams)[a]	% Evaluations Considered Comprehensive[b]
TABLE 3-26. Evaluating Abdominal Pain					
Hospital					
	29	4/15	11/29	20/29	17/29
	31	4/17	4/31	26/31	9/31
	36	4/26	7/36	19/36	27/36
	39	7/26	7/39	32/39	28/39
	135	19/84	29/135	97/135	81/135
		23%	21%	72%	60%

[a]Serial examinations documented via EMR or in free text.
[b] Comprehensive: Evaluation including more than one laboratory samples and imaging.

Documentation of serial examinations/reevaluations was 72%. Serial examinations are supported by the literature as an aid in diagnosis and disposition of the patient, and can be considered a valued method to address further pain control and patient satisfaction. A higher frequency of reevaluation will be encouraged.

Recommendations
- Increase frequency of gynecological and guaiac examinations.
- Increase frequency of serial examinations.

Section Three: High-Risk Patients (Table 3-27)
General Data: In general, the physicians should be commended for identifying and aggressively evaluating the high-risk patient population. The data support that the high-risk patient is being identified and clinically well-considered in the EDs. Literature identifies these patients, age >55 and/or with vascular or immunocompromising diseases, when presenting with APUE, as having significantly increased morbidity and mortality. This review also reflects the literature; high-risk patients were twice as likely to return to the ED, and four times as likely to be admitted on return. Physicians provided more comprehensive evaluations of the high-risk patients, including increased frequency of guaiac and CT studies, ECG review, and serial evaluations. Follow-up in <2 days was recommended more frequently than in low-risk patients. It could be advocated that these patients should return to the ED especially, considering the high frequency of admission, risk of pathology, and accessibility to further imaging studies, testing, and consultation.

Imaging with high-risk patients was frequent. Twenty-one percent of high-risk patients had two or more imaging studies in comparison to 4% in low-risk patients. This supports the thoroughness of the evaluation in high-risk patients.

Recommendations
- Maintain and/or increase the comprehensive examinations in all high-risk patients.
- Increase the recommendation of return in <2 days for reevaluation in high-risk patients.

Section Four: Common Missed Diagnoses (Table 3-28)
General Data: Per the first section, there were no documented "common missed diagnoses" in this study. This may be due to the study's small volume as the frequency of high-risk patients is probably adequate. Consideration of appendicitis in all patients was 38%. Consideration was probably underdocumented as was the past surgical history. Seventy-nine percent of females within reproductive age had pregnancy testing documented. This perhaps represents a significant risk in management, both from the possibility of ectopic pregnancy in the APUE patient, and from medicine provision and the uncertainty of

■ TABLE 3-27. High-Risk Patients

Hospital	No. Patients	% "High-Risk" Pts[a]	% HRPt With guaiac	% HRPt With CT	% HRPt With ECG	% HRPt With Documented Reevals (Serial Exams)[b]	% Evaluations of HRPt Considered Comprehensive[c]	% HRPt Returned to ED	No. HRPts Admitted on Return to ED	No. HRPts With Dx Common Dx Missed[d]
	29	9/29	6/9	3/9	4/9	7/9	6/9	3/9 (7/29)	1	0
	31	8/31	2/8	3/8	3/8	8/8	6/8	2/8 (5/31)	0	0
	36	11/36	3/11	7/11	2/11	10/11	9/11	0/11 (5/36)	0	0
na	39	11/39	5/11	7/11	2/11	10/11	11/11	3/11 (8/39)]	2	0
	135	39/135	16/39	20/39	11/39	35/39	32/39	8/39	3/39	0/39
		29%	41%	51%	28%	90%	82%	21%	8%	
Low risk			13/96	33/96	5/96	62/96	49/96	10/96	2/96	
			14%	34%	5%	65%	51%	10%	2%	

[a]High-risk pts (HRPt) = age >55 and/or significant PMHx.
[b]Serial exams documented via EMR or in free text.
[c]Comprehensive: Evaluation including more than one laboratory samples and imaging.
[d]AAA, appy, EP, MI, diverticulitis, perf viscus, mesenteric ischemia, bowel obstruction
Close Follow-up: 19/39 (49%) HRPt given <2-day follow-up instructions (37/96 [39%]).
Imaging in HRPt: 26/39 (67%) had KUB, CT, or US, and 8/39 (21%) had two or more imaging studies.
Imaging in non-HRPt: 52/96 (54%) had KUB, CT, or US, and 4/96 (4%) had two or more imaging studies.

■ TABLE 3-28. Common Missed Diagnoses

Hospital	No. Patients	% HRPt HTNive Pt With Imaging (R/O AAA)	% Pts w/ Consideration in DDx or Eval for (Appy)[a]	% Females <55 With Preg Test[b] (Ectopic Preg)	% HRPt With ECG and/or Cardiac Eval (MI)
	29	1/3	8/25	9/11	4/9
	31	1/3	10/30	10/12	4/8
	36	0/0	21/36	22/26	2/11
	39	3/6	12/39	11/17	2/11
	na				
	135	4/12	51/135	52/66	12/39
		33%	38%	79%	31%

[a]Documented in EMR diff Dx or in free text.
[b]Unless hyst documented.

pregnancy/fetal effects. About one-third of high-risk patients had an ECG and/ or cardiac enzymes for the consideration of a cardiac etiology. As pregnancy testing and ECGs are obtained efficiently and low cost, increased use will be encouraged.

Recommendations
- Increase frequency of consideration of appendicitis.
- Increase frequency of pregnancy testing.
- Increase frequency of cardiac evaluation in high-risk patients with APUE.

Section Five: Pain Control (Table 3-29)
General Data: Fifty percent of patients received pain medication. Only 4% received the medication prior to the MD evaluation. The article "Administration of Analgesia for Acute Abdominal Pain Sufferers in the Accident and Emergency Setting" (*Eur J Emerg Med*. December 2004;11(6):309-312) documented an average waiting time for analgesia of almost 90 minutes. An effort to address earlier medication to improve patient satisfaction and to improve the clinical evaluation is warranted. Also apparent within the review was that the pain scale was under-utilized for documentation of pain management.

Recommendations
- Emphasize on earlier pain medication administration. Address blockage in this process: physician access by RN, policy of sequential behavior—evaluation then treatment, rather than parallel management.
- Increase frequency of documentation of status post medication.

■ TABLE 3-29. Pain Control

Hospital	No. Patients	% Pts Given Pain Control	No. Pts Given Pain Control Prior to MD Eval	% Pts Given Narcotic for Pain Relief	% Positive Reduction in Pain Level Postmedication
	29	17/29	0	16/17	8/17
	31	12/31	1	10/12	5/12
	36	19/36	0	17/19	19/19
	39	20/39	2	17/20	15/20
	na				
	135	68/135	3/68	60/68	47/68
		50%	4%	88%	69%

Example of Data Collection Sheet

Quarterly Review—Abdominal Pain, Unclear Etiology

Quality Committee

Institution:

Physician #_____   Patient MR#_____

Patient age: <55   >55   Female   Male

Start of eval time (T chart time):_____

VS: WNL   HR   RR   SBP   T >38°;
                             >90   >20   <90   <36°

PMX: HTN   DM

                      ESRD   ESLD   Steriod HIV
                                     Depdt

Pain Control: Narcotic   NSAID   Other_____

            Pain control provided prior to eval by MD?   Y   N

            Effective? (RN noting lower number on pain scale)   Y   N

Exam: Stool Guiac?   Y   N

                             Pelvic or Bimanual?   Y   N

Ancillary Testing (circle all):

            Labs: CBC   CMP   Lipase Coags Cardiac

            Urine: CC   MC

                             Udip   U/A   Upreg

(Continued)

	ECG			
	KUB	Obst Series		
	CT:	Abdo& Pelvis	Renal	Other:_____ _____
	U/S:	Abdo.	RUQ	Pelvic

MDM/DDX:

	Specifics considered (written)	Appy	AAA	ACS/MI
	Reevaluation of pain noted?	Y	N	

Disposition:

	D/C'd	Time (T chart):_____	
	1° Dx:	AP, Unk Cause	Other:_____
	Follow-up:	No direction	<2 days Other:_____

Returns to LHS:

	<2 days	>2 days	No return
	Dx:_____		
	Comments:_____		
	Admit	D/C	

Reviewer Comments:

	Documentation: Minimal Poor Comprehensive	
	Evaluation consistent with pain/ presentation?	Y N
	Comments:_____	
	Pain management adequate?	Y N

(RN noting ↓ in pain #; or MD or RN comments indicating improvement)

	Disposition appropriate to pain level?	Y N
	Comments:_____	

Other:_____
_____
_____
_____

Conclusion

This was the first study of its kind on physician practice with abdominal pain patients; valuable data were isolated to assist the Quality Committee in providing focused feedback to the physicians in efforts to improve the high quality of care currently being provided. Further discussion and monitoring of the practice on this focused patient population will be encouraged.

Anthony Ferroggiaro, MD
Director of Quality

SEIZURE FOCUSED REVIEW

Quality Committee

Summary

Author's comments

This was an audit associated with a high-frequency presentation. Notable about the audit was the use of accepted standards as the ACEP clinical policies. These policies have been modified since the audit but largely the data present is still representative of expected management.

This audit also has utilization embedded within it. CT imaging has known impact on LOS and ED operational success as well and patient risk with radiation. Groups would do well to initiate tracking of CT imaging per physician and provide feedback.

Also included in this audit is community risk. Seizure activity is one clinical situation in which the laws prohibit use of motor vehicles. This audit reviews the compliance with the reporting aspect of the law.

Introduction

The Seizure Focused Review is a retrospective review of seizure management within the emergency departments in the health system.

The goals of this study were to assess the ED care provided to two populations based on evidence-based policies—first-time seizures and recurrent seizures. This was not a review of pediatric seizures or alcohol-related seizures. A future review will evaluate management of pediatric seizures.

The QC Committee has endorsed the ACEP clinical policies as standards of care for the practice of emergency medicine in the health system. The specific policies used in this study as a basis for evaluation were

- ACEP Practice Parameter: Neuroimaging in the Emergency Patient Presenting With Seizure.[54]

- ACEP Clinical Policy: Critical Issues in the Evaluation and Management of Adult Patients Presenting to the Emergency Department With Seizures.[55]

- ACEP Clinical Policy for the Initial Approach to Patients Presenting With a Chief Complaint of Seizure Who Are Not in Status Epilepticus.[56]

These policies can be obtained from the ACEP Web site.

Executive Summary and Recommendations

1. Excellent care was provided at all sites.
2. High acuity is represented.
    i. High admission rate may be appropriate based on clinical presentation and ED course.
        1. 92% for new onset seizures
        2. 73% for recurrent seizures
3. One discharged patient in 12 (8%) returned within 72 hours for recurrent seizures and this patient was determined to be noncompliant with medications.
4. Computed tomography (head) had high use
    a. High capture with new onset seizure patients (+MRI = 100%)
        i. Appropriate for subsequent care and current limited referral climate
    b. High CT use in recurrent seizure patients (60%)
        i. In background of high acuity this seems appropriate due to the frequency of new findings (16%)
    c. ACEP recommended indications were noted in 88% of patients receiving CT.
5. Utilization
    a. CMP (Na) and serum glucose evaluations were appropriately frequent (93%)
    b. CBC testing (85%)
        i. Overused in seizure patients
            1. The ED physician should review appropriateness with each laboratory request.
                a. Consider the significant laboratory TAT and that any test may require increased LOS and less efficiency in the ED with minimal ED clinical value.
                b. Goal: reduction by 50%.
        ii. Higher acuity/more medical complexity and less specific or classic presentations may support a CBC in general evaluations.
6. "Do not drive" recommendation (83%)
    a. Emphasis to increase frequency
        i. Goal is 100% compliance.
        ii. EMR is a simple, efficient mechanism for compliance.
            1. Increase the use of "additional instructions" which has the "do not drive" recommendation.
    b. State law information
        i. The ED MD has the responsibility to report the patient to the DMV if the patient does not have a primary care physician/neurologist.
            1. One patient in 10 did not have a PCP to refer back to and DMV was not notified.

Complete Summary
Demographics/Acuity (Tables 3-30 and 3-31)
A total of 65 patient cases were reviewed: 24 patients in the new-onset seizure group and 41 patients in the recurrent seizure group. Nineteen and 29 physicians' practices were reviewed, respectively.

It may be concluded that a high acuity population of seizure patients is represented in this review as the admission rate for new onset seizure patients was 92% and 73% in recurrent seizure patients. These high rates were due to the more complex presentations, associated illnesses/comorbidities in these patients, as well as nonreassuring ED courses. The ACEP Clinical Policy supports this admission rate as: "All patients with persistent abnormalities in mental status or examination should be admitted for further treatment." Indeed, individual case review identified frequent, persistent altered mental status as indication for inpatient placement.

Despite this high acuity and admission rates, 10 recurrent seizure patients and two new onset seizure patients were discharged from the EDs. Only one patient returned within 72 hours with recurrent seizures. This patient was found to have a continued low antiepileptic level and determined to be noncompliant with medications.

Head CT Review (Table 3-32)
The ACEP Clinical Policy for both new-onset and recurrent seizures:

Emergent NI (scan immediately) should be performed when a provider suspects a serious structural lesion. Clinical studies have shown a higher frequency of life-threatening lesions in patients with new focal deficits, persistent altered mental status (with or without intoxication), fever, recent trauma, persistent headache, history of cancer, history of anticoagulation, or suspicion of AIDS (Guideline).

Additionally, for patients with recurrent seizure (prior history of seizures) emergent NI should be considered if any of the following is (Option) (a) new seizure pattern or new seizure type, (b) prolonged postictal confusion or worsening mental status.

Urgent NI (scan appointment is included in the disposition or performed prior to disposition when follow-up of the patient's neurologic problem cannot be assured) should be performed for patients who have completely recovered from their seizure and for whom no clear-cut cause has been identified (eg, hypoglycemia, hyponatremia, tricyclic overdose) to help identify a possible structural cause. Because adequate follow-up is needed to ensure a patient's neurologic health, urgent NI may be obtained prior to disposition when timely follow-up cannot be assured (Option).

One hundred percent of new onset patients had CNS imaging on presentation/admission. All but one patient (MRI as inpatient) had an ED CT. Sixty percent of the recurrent seizure patients had CT imaging.

■ TABLE 3-30. New Onset Seizure

Hospital	No. Patients	No. MDs	CMP/Glu	CBC	Head CT	Tx: BZPD	Tx: Fos	Admit	DC on Anti Sz Med	Do Not Drive Inst	Return <72°
	4	3	4/4	4/4	4/4	3/4	3/4	4/4	na		
	8	5	7/8	7/8	7/8	2/8	1/8	8/8	na		
	2	2	2/2	2/2	2/2	0/2	2/2	2/2	na		
	9	8	9/9	9/9	9/9	6/9	5/9	7/9	2/2	2/2	0
	1	1	1/1	1/1	1/1	1/1	1/1	1/1	na		
Totals	**24**	**19**	**23/24**	**23/24**	**23/24**	**12/24**	**12/24**	**22/24**		**2/2**	**0**

XH: one patient not given meds but admit.

YH: one MRI not CT; one CT deferred but admitted; low med rx.

ZH: one patient excused—etoh; no bzdp only fos given.

1H: one pt in DKA delirium; 2 pt started keppra, neurontin respectively after neurology consult in ED—both discharged home with no recurrence in 72 hours.

2H: one peds and four etoh excused.

Do not drive: Original draft—data were 4/10—revised to new onset 2/2 and recurrent 8/10—difficulty with abstraction of the data due to the EMR not retaining all of the EMR "Additional Instructions" within which for the seizure Dx include the directive not to drive.

DMV: Currently state law requires ED MD notification if the patient does not have a primary care physician—it is unclear if this extends to county clinic patients, etc. The DMV indicator has been removed as a standard.

■ TABLE 3-31. Recurrent Seizure

Hospital	No. Patients	No. MDs	CMP/Glu	CBC	Anti Sz Level	Head CT	Tx: BZPD	Tx: Fos	D/C	Docu Indication for Recurrence	Do Not Drive Inst	Return <72°
	9	5	8/9	6/9	6/9	7/9	4/9	5/9	3/9	3/3	2/3	1
	15	10	14/15	12/15	6/15	7/15	5/15	5/15	5/15	4/5	5/5	0
	2	1	2/2	2/2	2/2	2/2	2/2	2/2	0/2	na		
	11	9	10/11	9/11	8/8	6/11	6/11	6/11	2/11	2/2	1/2	0
	4	4	3/4	3/4	3/3	3/4	1/4	2/4	0/4	na		
TOTALS	**41**	**29**	**37/41**	**32/41**	**25/41**	**25/41**	**18/41**	**20/41**	**10/41**	**9/10**	**8/10**	**1**

XH: sz levels: one pt not rx on valproate; one antisz med—keppra; 2 pts not on meds—no levels checked; CTs—2 pts not indicated—same pattern of sz; 3 pt d/c—recurrence due to low dil level; returned pt with recurrent sz—cont'd noncompliance.

YH: one pt no BS check; sz levels—one pt dil tox; 5 pt d/c'd—0 had head CT, no returns; one pt on depakote—no additional anti-sz med.

ZH: both CT—new sz pattern; one pt bzdp infusion for status; both pt admit.

1H: 3 pt no sz med levels—one neurontin, one not started dil, one off dil for one mo.; no rx—one on teg; both doc indic rec—low levels.

2H: one pt not on med no level check.

■ TABLE 3-32. Head CT Review

Hospital No. Patients	New Onset + ED CT	If CT Def; Pt Return <72°	Recurrent Sz + ED CT	Indic: Concern for IC process	Indic: CHI, Ca, Immuno	Indic: Fever	Indic: Persist HA	Indic: Anticoag	Indic: Focal	Indic: >40 years	Indic: New Pattern	Changes on CT (New [Old])
13	4/4	na	7/9	a	a, b		c	c, d, e			e, f	1 [4]
23	7/8	na	7/15	a, b, c, d, e		e	f				g, h	4 [3]
4	2/2	na	2/2	a							a, b	0 [2]
20	9/9	na	6/11	a		b	b	c	c	d, e	d, e	1 [7]
5	1/1	na	3/4						a, b		a	2 [1]
TOTALS 65	23/24	na	25/41									8/48
	96%		60%									25/48

New onset sz and ED CT: YH—CT deferred in ED and pt admitted.
Total CT: 48/65 = 74%.
16% (8/48) were new findings on CT; 52% (25/48) had abnormal CT studies.
Letters represent individual patients—some patients had more than one indication for imaging.
16% (4/25) of recurrent seizure patients had new findings on CT.

Twenty-two of 25 patients with recurrent seizures who subsequently received ED CT imaging had documented courses and indications for imaging based on the ACEP Clinical Policy recommendations. Sixteen percent of all recurrent seizure patients receiving a head CT had new findings, including metastatic tumors and intracranial hemorrhage. One hundred percent imaging was obtained in patients with known coagulopathy and seizure activity.

Fifty-two percent of all patients receiving a head CT had abnormal findings on the examination (atrophy, old infarction, encephalomalacia).

It can be concluded that this high usage of imaging is appropriate and proper based on clinical presentation/suspicion and this high acuity population.

Laboratory Usage

Serum sodium and glucose levels were determined in 93% patients. Only two patients were determined hypoglycemic, identified in either the prehospital setting or the ED, and both were admitted.

CBC usage was 85% (55/65). There is limited to no direct benefit in the CBC value in the specific evaluation for the etiology of new onset or recurrent seizures. In consideration of this high usage, as stated above, this population of seizure patients had extensive comorbidities encouraging a more thorough understanding of medical status and to assist in the ongoing management postadmission.

Discharge Instructions

Ten of 12 patients who were discharged from the EDs were instructed in writing not to drive. It should be noted that the Additional Instructions section provided in the "recurrent seizure" and "new-onset seizure" EMR discharge instructions easily fulfills this safety recommendation. Physicians should be encouraged to include the "Additional instructions" within the discharge instructions provided to the patients. It should also be verbally reinforced by staff upon discharge.

The state law requires ED MDs to report active/uncontrolled seizure patients to the DMV *if the patient does not have a primary care provider.* All of the discharged patients were discharged from hospitals. Nine of 10 patients were referred back to their primary care physician, clinic, or neurologist. Of the two patients referred to outpatient clinics, one patient was established.

Anthony Ferroggiaro, MD

CENTRAL VENOUS CATHETER AUDIT

Quality Committee

Author's comments

This was a comprehensive intervention including the promotion of new technology within the EDs, the organization of training sessions as interventions, the advocacy of US equipment purchase to the health system, the promotion of a US "guru" as champion and addressing a national patient safety goal of reducing CVC infection rates (CLABSI). Challenges to this audit were with the definition of complication and the advocacy of a threshold of practice that would trigger review training. As noted within the text, the definition of complication was any additional needle stick after the first and this "high" threshold was based on the patient's perspective. It has been observed that US use with CVC insertion reduced the number of needle insertions. Certainly this threshold could be debated within the physician group and a local standard could be inserted.

The "proposed threshold for CVC procedural competency" is a big policy jump. To the author's knowledge there is no requirement nationally or locally or any literature about this type of policy/threshold. But there should be. Practice is essential to success, and it should be the organization's responsibility to ensure a physician's success with a policy or requirement for significant procedures and a means (with best EBM) to provide practice and feedback for the physician. There are patterns of this idea within the medical literature. The first example is debate within the AHA/ACC on frequency of cardiac catheterizations and PTCA success resulting in an advocated threshold but also an acknowledgment of a lack of data. The second example is the article by Youngquist et al. on paramedic success with pediatric intubation identifying a skill atrophy pattern over time and risk issue.[57] Perhaps some brave academic EM physician will find opportunity to create a national reporting program and achieve some publications to clarify this topic!

Executive summary of CVC audit
Complications

- 14% Complication rate (233 cases reviewed).
  - Majority of complications were failure of access.
  - No pneumothoraces were identified.
- Divisions varied in complication rate.
  - 4% to 32%

Volume and Competency

- No statistical association can be made between annual volume of CVC per MD and competency due to limited data.
  - Physicians and sites of higher frequency and volume of CVCs had fewer complications.
- In an effort to define a reasonable benchmark, addressing the variability in volume and competency, and to support the physicians, calculations were conducted.

Ultrasound

- Ultrasound activity with CVC placement appears *to increase* CVC complication rate
- One division had high rate of complications with US use.

Possible Actions

- Some potential actions:
  - Authorization or rejection of the proposed benchmark for assessing competency with CVC placement as defined by the data (see above).
    - Data support annual mark of three CVC procedures per MD. This proposed benchmark could be used as a threshold such that physicians completing less than three CVC procedures annually would attend a procedural review session
  - To address the complication rate and low volume–induced procedural competency, education could develop a review course including procedure video review, simulation lab activity, and US practice with CVC placement. Alternatively, medical directors could address complications within divisions.
  - A 5% divisional complication goal could be proposed. This would provide a target for educational intervention and yearly data comparison.
  - Development of a departmental US group that could centralize the divisional activity of US introduction, credentialing, and maintenance of competency.

Introduction

This is the first procedural audit for the group. Future procedural audits will include lumbar puncture and intubation procedures. These three procedures will receive focus due to high frequency and high risk within emergency medicine.

Reviewing the CVC activity represents a unique opportunity with the introduction of US to all EDs, the concurrent development of a CVC Guideline, and ongoing quality approach of providing feedback to colleagues and support of excellent care.

Methods

The initial database was obtained from the billing company and consisted of basic data output using CPT codes for CVC. A chart review and audit tool was developed and two researchers/scribes completed the individual case review via EMR. Questions on the audit tool were formatted from CVC Guideline and literature review.

Two hundred thirty three events were reviewed. All divisions are represented. Fifty-four physicians were reviewed. Entry data and relationship assessment were managed via Microsoft Access.

Several physicians worked at multiple sites. The combined data were attributed once and to the major site—the site of the majority of patients evaluated by the physician.

MDs were excluded from review if they had <250 patients seen over 12 months unless the MD had completed CVC procedure.

In this review a complication is defined through the patient's eyes. It is a failure to access on first attempt requiring movement to another access site or termination of the procedure without second attempt, resulting in no CVC placement and/or injury with any attempt.

Patients requiring *CPR* were identified in the EMR record. *Respiratory distress* was indicated if the MD or the presentation indicated that the patient could not be laid flat for line placement. Key words identified were: severe respiratory distress (not just severe distress), oxygen saturation was <90%, unresponsive or combination of such. If the patient was intubated prior to CVC placement, the indication for femoral line due to respiratory distress was nullified. Consideration for a *compressible site* should be supported with data or in the presentation such as bleeding pattern and/or the index of INR >2.

Results

There were 233 CVC placements reviewed out of 112,969 opportunities (the calculated volume of patients presenting to all EDs during this time frame). This represented a frequency of 0.21% (Table 3-33). *This rate could be used as one factor in the comparison of acuity between emergency departments.* There was a wide variance in activity between sites with a range (0.09% to 0.44%) and a wide variance in activity within physicians with some MDs completing zero CVCs in the year evaluated (Figure 3-24).

Femoral venous CVC access occurred in 64% of the placements with the subclavian venous access (24%) and the internal jugular venous access (12%) being the other two options (Figure 3-25).

Complications

There were 33 complications documented for the 233 placements (14%) (Figure 3-26). The majority of the complications were due to failure to access (28/33 [85%]), either requiring no CVC placement or a decision to attempt a second site. There were no hematomas and no pneumothoraces documented in this group of patients. The attempts to access the left femoral vein resulted in the highest frequency of complications with the attempts to access the right internal jugular vein having the fewest (Table 3-34). Of the thoracic attempts, either

■ TABLE 3-33. Average Rate of Insertion			
Site	Number of CVCs Placed in 20XX	Adult Volume of Each Site	# CVC per 1 Opportunity
H1	95	20,556	0.0046
H2	55	19,958	0.0028
H3	21	24,376	0.0009
H4	25	26,500	0.0009
H5	37	21,579	0.0017
Totals	233	112,969	0.0021

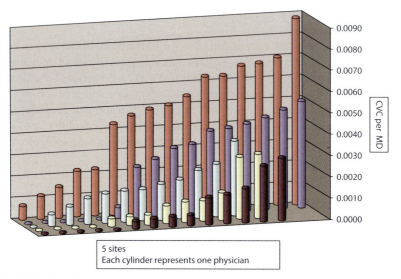

FIGURE 3-24. CVC placement activity for all divisions.

internal jugular or subclavian vein CVC, a postattempt/placement CXR was documented in 92% to 100% attempts dependent on the site (data not shown).

There was great variance in complication rates per division though the data may be skewed by volume of activity. There was a trend toward fewer complications at certain divisions and notably these sites had higher frequency of placement. Two

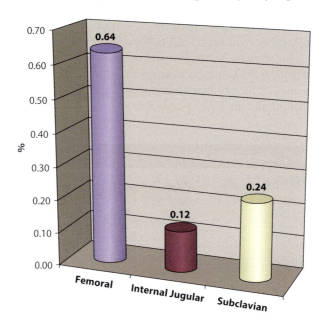

FIGURE 3-25. CVC placement frequency per vascular site.

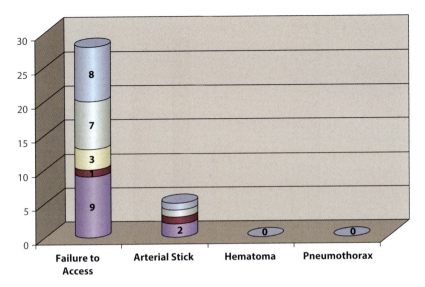

FIGURE 3-26. Types of complications.

divisions had nearly double the average complication rate for the total chart population (Figure 3-27). As per Figure 3-28, the frequency of complications was associated with the number of procedures completed. There is a trend toward fewer complications when higher numbers of CVCs are completed annually though the underpowered study limits statistical association.

As shown in Table 3-35, one division CVC placement data are provided. All divisions have similar data compilation and these data have been provided to the respective medical directors. Several MDs had complications (MDs 2, 4, and 9) and these MDs will receive feedback on their data including patient MR numbers in order to review their patient charts. All physicians with complications will be requested to participate in a CVC-US guidance educational course in order to

■ **TABLE 3-34.** Complications per Opportunities Dependent on Site of CVC Insertion

Site	Events	Opportunities	%
L Fem	9	36	0.25
R Fem	12	116	0.10
L IJ	1	5	0.20
R IJ	2	24	0.08
L SC	1	10	0.10
R SC	8	46	0.17
	33	**237**	

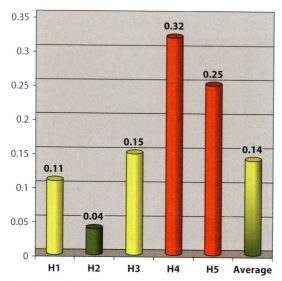

FIGURE 3-27. Rate of complications.

review technique. Several physicians will be acknowledged for high volume and no complications.

Ultrasound Use

The use of ultrasound at each division was also reviewed (data not shown). Only three of five divisions at the time of this audit had US equipment present in the ED

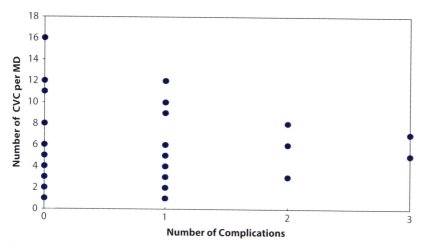

FIGURE 3-28. Complications per number of CVCs per MD annually.

■ **TABLE 3-35.** Description of Complications per Physician (One Division)

Physician Name	Pt MR	Venous Site	US Guidance	CVC ED Complications	CXR: Good Cath. Position
MD1		R femoral	False	Failure to Access	na (fem)
		R subclavian	False	None	Yes
MD2		L femoral	False	None	na (fem)
		L femoral	False	None	na (fem)
		R femoral	False	Failure to Access	na (fem)
		R femoral	False	Failure to access	na (fem)
		L femoral	False	None	na (fem)
		L femoral	False	Failure to access	na (fem)
		R femoral	False	None	na (fem)
MD3		R femoral	False	None	na (fem)
			False		
		R int jugular	False	None	No
			False		
MD4		R subclavian	False	None	Yes
		R subclavian	False	None	Yes
		L subclavian	False	Arterial stick	Yes
		L subclavian	False	None	Yes
		R femoral	False	None	na (fem)
		R femoral	False	Failure to access	
MD5		R subclavian	False	None	Yes
MD6		L subclavian	False	None	Yes
		L subclavian	False	None	No
MD7		L femoral	False	None	na (fem)
MD8		R subclavian	False	None	No
MD9		R int jugular	False	None	No
		R subclavian	False	Failure to access	
		R femoral	False	Failure to access	na (fem)

for use with CVC insertion. Of these three divisions, US was used in 11% (24/212) of the insertions. With attempts at internal jugular vein access, the US was used in greater than 57% of attempts whereas in femoral venous access it was used in only 7% of the attempts.

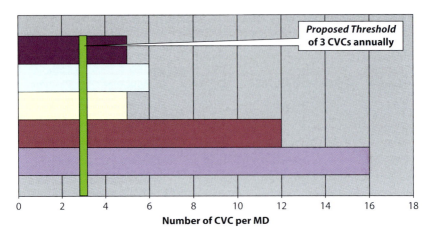

FIGURE 3-29. Divisional (5) physician range of CVC insertion as justification for proposed CVC insertion benchmark.

Proposed Threshold for CVC Procedural Competency

With the above data and considering the average annual number of patients managed (separate data), we were able to calculate an expected average number of CVC insertions annually for all physicians. The result was *three CVCs annually (3.18 + SD 6.52) per MD.* This rate can be a reasonable benchmark for the physicians in the group for maintaining competency. One physician at every division has achieved a number of CVCs beyond the threshold when working regularly; thus, each division and physician has potential volume to achieve threshold (Figure 3-29).

Conclusions

Possible Actions

- Authorization or rejection of the proposed benchmark for assessing competency with CVC placement as defined by the data (see above).
  - The data support an annual mark of three CVC procedures per MD. This proposed benchmark could be used as a threshold such that physicians completing less than three CVC procedures annually would attend a procedural review session and/or arrange for other technique review.
- To address the complication rate and low volume induced procedural competency, education could develop a review course including procedure video review, simulation lab activity, and US practice with CVC placement. Alternatively, medical directors could address complications within divisions.
- A 5% divisional complication goal could be proposed. This would provide a target for educational intervention and yearly data comparison.
- Development of a departmental US group that could centralize the divisional activity of US introduction, credentialing, and maintenance of competency.

CENTRAL VENOUS CATHETER LIFE SPAN AUDIT

Placement in the Emergency Department CVC to ICU Management

Author's comments

This subaudit was a result of the prior CVC audit as access to the subsequent life span of the CVC was through the EMR.

As per the introduction, the ED MD has an impact on the continuity of care of the hospitalized patient. With publishing these data, emphasis was placed on the value of methods of CVC insertion and the reliance of subsequent services on high-quality ED care. As the reader is well aware, CLABSIs are a focus of hospitals since the CMS focuses on this as an outcome measure.

These data were supported by the published study by LeMaster.[58]

There is political value (and danger) in these data. The value will be in reaffirming the significant effect of EM care on the patient beyond the borders and time period within the ED with emphasis on the known value that the ED has on reducing hospital LOS and cost. The danger would be a challenging interaction with the ICU-based physicians.

Introduction

This brief report is one arm of the CVC audit which has been completed on all CVC placements at the five ED divisions in the health system.

Reviewing the CVC activity represented a unique opportunity as CVC placement is a high-frequency practice within the system and, in general, is high risk to the patient; the study would be concurrent with the introduction of US to all EDs. There was also a concurrent development of a CVC Guideline, and ongoing quality approach of providing feedback to colleagues and support of excellent care.

Methods

The initial database was obtained from our billing company and consisted of basic demographic output using CPT codes for CVC. A chart review and audit tool was developed and two researchers/scribes completed the individual case review via EMR. Questions on the audit tool were formatted from CVC Guideline and literature review.

Two hundred thirty three events were reviewed. All divisions are represented. Fifty-four physicians were reviewed. Entry data and relationship assessment were managed via Microsoft Access.

For data abstraction, the determination of the CVC placement time was according to a hierarchy of charting areas and personnel. The primary time was the time noted in the ED text/MDM/progress of the EMR during the patient's ED management. A secondary time (if no primary time noted) was the time of the EMR closure if the chart was closed within 4-6 hours of ED entry indicating a window in which the CVC was placed as this represents the last note in the ED EMR prior to patient transfer to the floor. The third time was the first RN entry in ICU central-line documentation. The determination of the removal time was the last RN entry in ICU central-line documentation indicating line removed.

Results

One hundred ninety five charts of 233 had placement and removal time data (Figure 3-30). The average life span of an ED-placed CVC was 90.3 hours (range 2.2-563.8 hours) which represented a mean 3.8 days (range 0.09-23.5 days).

The first quartile maximum life span was 1.3 days; the second quartile was 2.9 days; and the third quartile was 5.6 days. Thus over 75% of ED-placed CVC were removed before 6 days with an average life span of 2.3 days for the three quartiles.

Table 3-36 shows the nine cases that had CVC life spans greater than 10 days. Notable is that five sites were the femoral vein in this grouping.

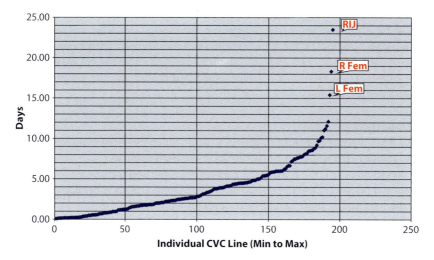

FIGURE 3-30. Emergency department placed CVC life span in ICU.

TABLE 3-36. Nine Patients With Longest CVC Life Span and Site of Access			
Patient Last Name	**MR#**	**Days**	**Site**
HE		23.5	R int jugular
PO		18.3	R femoral
AL		15.4	L femoral
ME		12.1	R int jugular
CL		11.6	R femoral
WA		11.2	R femoral
RO		11.0	L subclavian
SC		10.2	R Subclavian
LA		10.1	R Femoral

Discussion

These data are provided to the ICU team and the EM physicians in efforts toward joint quality goals. These data will have future impact on CVC site decision making by the EM physicians.

There are no specific thresholds, indeed there is a paucity of data on risk of complications and life span of the CVC. A general consideration is that with increased retention time within the patient will provide increased risk of complications.

Utilizing data provided through *infection control*, CVC placement patients were cross-referenced with BSI (bloodstream infection) events. Three cases were identified according to visit dates. Access site correspondence was two femoral sites and one internal jugular site. Life span was 9.8 and 6 days for two of three cases; one further study did not have data for abstraction. None of the nine longest life span CVC patients had documented BSI.

The prior CVC audit identified that 64% of ED CVC placements used the femoral venous site. It is well acknowledged in the literature that femoral access sites have a higher rate of infectious and thrombotic complications. Efforts are being made to assist the evolution of ED CVC practice using US-guidance for placement, reviewing procedural quality, and advocacy of nonfemoral vein placements. These data will reinforce the value in nonfemoral site selection.

Based on the data, other than modifying the site selection within the ED, there are opportunities for quality improvement. One opportunity would be for the ICU team to establish an acceptable threshold for CVC retention. The data may provide base for this discussion. This discussion would need to recognize the variables of cost of replacement in personnel hours and equipment and balance this with patient safety.

The distribution plot of the CVC life span data (end) has been conveniently distributed into quartiles with the 150-200 section being most dramatic in life span period. Clearly this is a most opportune area for quality management with program/threshold development.

Another opportunity would be for the ICU team to consider a program to evaluate central lines for "justifiable" treatment or removal. Gowardman et al. provided an interesting study to this topic in which a removal policy was introduced to remove the CVC on ICU discharge. The results were lower CVC in situ times when policy was followed (5.1 vs 8.1 days), low CVC reinsertion rates (7%), and no difference in incidence of bloodstream infections between the groups.[59]

Both EM physicians and ICU teams could find opportunity for practice review based on the above data. Moreover, a joint quality effort would likely provide greater quality impact and could be considered.

Anthony Ferroggiaro, MD

REFERENCES

1. National Institute for Clinical Excellence. *Principles for best practice in clinical audit.* Abingdon, England: Radcliffe Medical Press, Ltd; 2002.

2. NICE. NICE National Institute for Health and Care Excellence. Retrieved from http://www.nice.org.uk/. October 10, 2014.

3. Berenson RA. Grading a physician's value - the misapplication of performance measurement. *N Engl J Med*. 2013;369(22):2079-2081.

4. Holmboe ES. Assessing quality of care. *JAMA*. 2008;299(3):338-340.

5. Werner RM, Bradlow ET. Relationship between Medicare's hospital compare performance measures and mortality rates. *JAMA*. 2006;296(22):2694-2702.

6. Pronovost PJ, Hudson DW. Improving healthcare quality through organisational peer-to-peer assessment: lessons from the nuclear power industry. *BMJ Qual Saf*. 2012;21(10):872-875.

7. Hoekstra JW, Pollack CV Jr, Roe MT, et al. Improving the care of patients with non-ST-elevation acute coronary syndromes in the emergency department: the CRUSADE initiative. *Acad Emerg Med*. 2002;9(11):1146-1155.

8. CMS. About hospital compare. Medicare.gov. Retrieved from http://www.medicare.gov/hospitalcompare/About/What-Is-HOS.html. September 5, 2014.

9. Smulowitz PB, O'Malley J. Increased use of the emergency department after health care reform in Massachusetts. *Ann Emerg Med*. 2014;64(2):107-115.

10. Pitts SR, Pines JM. National trends in emergency department occupancy, 2001 to 2008: effect of inpatient admissions versus emergency department practice intensity. *Ann Emerg Med*. 2012;60(6):679-686.

11. Goodacre SW. Point-of-care testing may reduce length of stay but not emergency department crowding. *Ann Emerg Med*. 2013;61(2):153-154.

12. Kocher KE, Meurer WJ. Effect of testing and treatment on emergency department length of stay using a national database. *Acad Emerg Med*. 2012;19(5):525-534.

13. Hoot N. Systematic review of emergency department crowding: causes, effects, and solutions. *Ann Emerg Med*. 2008;52(2):126-136.

14. Mason S, Weber EJ. Time patients spend in the emergency department: England's 4-hour rule—a case of hitting the target but Missing the Point? *Ann Emerg Med*. 2012;341-349.

15. Abualenain J, Frohna WJ. Emergency department physician-level and hospital-level variation in admission rates. *Ann Emerg Med*. 2013;61(6):638-643.

16. Nestler DM, Fratzke AR. Effect of a physician assistant as triage liaison provider on patient throughput in an academic emergency department. *Acad Emerg Med*. 2012;19(11):1235-1241.

17. Wiler JL, Rooks SP. Update on midlevel provider utilization in U.S. emergency departments, 2006 to 2009. *Acad Emerg Med*. 2012;19(8):986-989.

18. Porter ME, Teisberg EO. *Redefining health care*. Boston, MA: Harvard Business School Press; 2006.

19. Mittiga M R. The spectrum and frequency of critical procedures performed in a pediatric emergency department: implications of a provider level view. *Ann of Emerg Med*. 2013;61(3):263-270.

20. Sackles JC. The importance of first pass success when performing orotracheal intubation in the emergency department. *Acad Emerg Med*. 2013;20(1):71-78.

21. Porter ME. What is value in health care? *N Engl J Med*. 2010;363:2477-2481.

22. Donabedian A. Evaluating the quality of medical care. *Milbank Q*. 2005;83(4):691-729.

23. CDC. Ambulatory health care data. National Center for Healthcare Statistics. Retrieved from http://www.cdc.gov/nchs/ahcd.htm. October 6, 2014.

24. Ransom ER. *The healthcare quality book*. Chicago, IL: Health Administration Press; 2008.

25. Wyer PC. Responsiveness to change: a quality indicator for assessment of knowledge translation systems. *Acad Emerg Med*. 2007;14(11):928-930.

26. Ivers N, Jamtvedt G, Flottorp S, Young JM. Audit and feedback: effects on professional practice and healthcare outcomes. *Cochrane Database Syst Rev*. 2012;6. doi:10.1002/14651858.

27. Choudhry NK. Systematic review: the relationship between clinical experience and quality of health care. *Ann Intern Med*. 2005;142(4):260-273.

28. Pusic MV, Kessler D. Experience curves as an organizing framework for deliberate practice in emergency medicine learning. *Acad Emerg Med*. 2012;19(12): 1476-1480.

29. Youngquist ST, Henderson DT. Paramedic self-efficacy and skill retention in pediatric airway management. *Acad Emerg Med*. 2008;15(12):1295-1303.

30. Kovacs G, Bullock G. A randomized controlled trial on the effect of educational interventions in promoting airway management skill maintenance. *Ann Emerg Med*. 2000;36(4):301-309.

31. Su E. A randomized controlled trial to assess decay in acquired knowledge among paramedics completing a pediatric resuscitation course. *Acad Emerg Med*. 2000;7(7):779-786.

32. Jamtvedt G, Young JM, Kristoffersen DT, O'Brien MA, Oxman AD. Does telling people what they have been doing change what they do? A systematic review of the effects of audit and feedback. *Qual Saf Health Care*. 2006;15(6):433-436.

33. Lang ES, Wyer PC, Haynes RB. Knowledge translation: closing the evidence-to-practice gap. *Ann Emerg Med*. 2007;49(3):355-363.

34. Grimshaw JM. Knowledge translation of research findings. *Implement Sci*. 2012;7(50):1-17.

35. Graham ID, Tetroe J. Some theoretical underpinnings of knowledge translation. *Acad Emerg Med*. 2007;14(11):936-941.

36. Davis D. Impact of formal continuing medical education. *JAMA*. 1999;282(9):869-874.

37. Dawson B, Trapp RG. *Basic and clinical biostatistics*. New York, NY: McGraw-Hill; 2004.

38. Hulley SB, Cummings SR. *Designing clinical research*. Baltimore, MD: Williams and Wilkins; 1988.

39. Berwick D. The science of improvement. *JAMA*. 2008;299(10):1182-1184.

40. Marsan RJ Jr, Shaver KJ, Sease KL, Shofer FS, Sites FD, Hollander JE. Evaluation of a clinical decision rule for young adult patients with chest pain. *Ann Emerg Med*. 2005;12(1):26-32.

41. Rivers M. Early goal-directed therapy in the treatment of severe sepsis and septic shock. *N Engl J Med*. 2001;345(19):1368-1377.

42. Crichlow A. Overuse of computed tomography pulmonary angiography in the evaluation of patients with suspected pulmonary embolism in the emergency department. *Acad Emerg Med*. 2012;19(11):1219-1226.

43. Venkatesh A. Evaluation of pulmonary embolism in the emergency department and consistency with a national quality measure: quantifying the opportunity for improvement. *Arch Intern Med*. 2012;172(13):1028-1032.

44. Penaloza A, Verschuren F. Comparison of the unstructured clinician Gestalt, the wells score, and the revised Geneva score to estimate pretest probability for suspected pulmonary embolism. *Ann Emerg Med.* 2013;62(2):117-124.

45. Gibler W. Practical implementation of the guidelines for unstable angina/non-ST-segment elevation myocardial infarction in the emergency department. *Ann Emerg Med.* 2005;46(2):185-197.

46. Boersma E, Pieper KS, Steyerberg EW. Predictors of outcome in patients with acute coronary syndromes without persistent ST-segment elevation: results from an international trial of 9461 patients. *Circulation.* 2000;101(22):2557-2567.

47. Ferguson JJ, Califf RM. Enoxaparin vs unfractionated heparin in high-risk patients with non–ST-segment elevation acute coronary syndromes managed with an intended early invasive strategy primary results of the SYNERGY randomized trial. *JAMA.* 2004;292(1):45-54.

48. Cohen M, Demers C. A comparison of low-molecular-weight heparin with unfractionated heparin for unstable coronary artery disease. *N Engl J Med.* 1997; 337(7):447-452.

49. Antman EM, McCabe CH, Gurfinkel EP, et al. Enoxaparin prevents death and cardiac ischemic events in unstable angina/non–Q-wave myocardial infarction : results of the thrombolysis in myocardial infarction (TIMI) 11B trial. *Circulation.* 1999;100(15):1593-1601.

50. Yusuf S, Fox K K. Effects of clopidogrel in addition to aspirin in patients with acute coronary syndromes without ST-segment elevation. *N Engl J Med.* 2001;345(7):494-502.

51. Fesmire F. Are we putting the cart ahead of the horse: who determines the standard of care for the management of patients in the emergency department? *Ann Emerg Med.* 2005;46(2):198-200.

52. Jain S, Cheng J, Alpern ER, et al. Management of febrile neonates in US pediatric emergency departments. *Pediatrics.* 2014;133(2):187-195.

53. ACEP. Clinical policy: critical issues for the initial evaluation and management of patients presenting with a chief complaint of nontraumatic acute abdominal pain. *Ann Emerg Med.* 2000;36(4):406-415.

54. ACEP. Practice parameter: neuroimaging in the emergency patient presenting with seizure. *Ann Emerg Med.* 1996;28(1):114-118.

55. ACEP. Clinical policy: critical issues in the evaluation and management of adult Patients presenting to the emergency department with seizures. *Ann Emerg Med.* 2014;43(5):605-625.

56. ACEP. Clinical policy for the initial approach to patients presenting with a chief complaint of seizure who are not in status epilepticus. *Ann Emerg Med.* 1997;29(5):706-724.

57. Youngquist S. Paramedic self-efficacy and skill retention in pediatric airway management. *Acad Emerg Med.* 2008;15(12):1295-1303.

58. LeMaster C. Infection and natural history of emergency department-placed central venous catheters. *Ann Emerg Med.* 2010;56(5):492-497.

59. Gowardman JR, Kelaher C, Whiting J. Impact of a formal removal policy for central venous catheters on duration of catheterisation. *Med J Aust.* 2005;182(5):249-250.

Assessment of Practice Performance

4A: The ABEM APP Patient Care Practice Improvement Requirement

- ■ **WHAT IS APP?**
- ■ **DOES THE APP PCPI REQUIREMENT ADD TO TECHNICAL QUALITY?**
- ■ **ATTESTATION**
- ■ **VERIFICATION OF ACTIVITY**
- ■ **EXAMPLES FOR COMPLIANCE WITH THE APP PCPI COMPONENT**

  Adult Seizure Management

  Seizure and Neuroimaging

  Adult Asymptomatic HTN Management

  Early Pregnancy

  Suspected Pulmonary Embolism

  Acute Abdominal Pain, Risk of Appendicitis

  Acute Headache

  Syncope

  Renal Colic

This chapter will be a brief introduction to one component of the American Board of Medical Specialties (ABMS) and American Board of Emergency Medicine (ABEM) Maintenance of Certification (MOC) requirement, the Assessment of Practice Performance, since it is aligned with the "hard quality" subject of this text. This chapter will describe the board certification requirement including the PCPI component of APP and provide specific discussion and an outline of the requirement for individual BC emergency physicians. Most importantly, the chapter will finish with examples and outlines of APP projects that could be used by a physician to complete the APP PCPI requirement. Chapter 4B will include a description of the APP Communication/Professionalism (C/P) component.

■ WHAT IS APP?

APP is one approach by the ABMS to encourage the application of the knowledge-based material (LLSA, etc) into clinical practice.[1] The assessment of practice performance is the fourth component of the ABMS continuous learning process, with licensure, LLSA testing, and the certification (or recertification) examination as the other components (Table 4a-1). The emphasis of the APP is on the application of the knowledge examined through the LLSA and examinations.

Part IV—Practice Performance Assessment

They are evaluated in their clinical practice according to specialty-specific standards for patient care. They are asked to demonstrate that they can assess the quality of care they provide compared to peers and national benchmarks and then apply the best evidence or consensus recommendations to improve that care using follow-up assessments.[2]

The two components of ABEM's APP are the Patient Care Practice Improvement activity (PCPI) and the Communication/Professionalism (C/P) patient feedback program. This section will focus on the PCPI activity as it meets the "hard quality" factor aligned with the author's goal of raising the value of clinical quality and performance as well as a consistency with the topics of Chapters 2 and 3.

Reviewing the ABEM Web site on APP, the requirements for PCPI activity will vary according to the board certification year and status of the physician. In general, the ABEM requires one PCPI activity over the first 5 years and a second over

---

■ TABLE 4A-1. Components of ABMS (ABEM) Continuous Learning Process

1. Licensure—continuous and inclusive of ongoing CME
2. LLSA testing
3. Certification (recertification)
4. Assessment of practice performance
   a. Patient care practice improvement activity
   b. Communication/professionalism

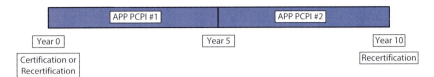

FIGURE 4A-1. General representation of APP PCPI activity and board certification.

the subsequent 5 years of the 10-year period between recertification (Figure 4a-1). A physician, when in doubt about his or her requirements, can easily log in to the ABEM Web site which has a well-formatted tracking system.

ABEM requires a standard process improvement format (similar to PDSA) when completing the activity:

> *Patient care practice improvement activities that meet ABEM requirements are focused on improving or maintaining clinical processes compared to established standards. ABEM requires that diplomates follow four basic steps when completing a PCPI activity. Those steps are* **measurement, comparison to standards, improvement, and evaluation of the improvement implemented.**[3]

Four basic steps are required (Figure 4a-2). A PCPI activity must include the following four steps[4]:

1. Review patient clinical care data from 10 of your patients. The data must be related to a single presentation, disease, or clinical care process that is

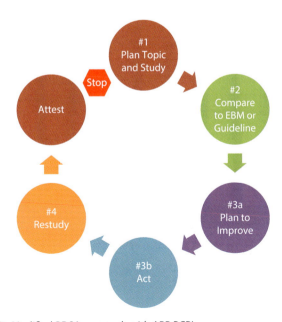

FIGURE 4A-2. Modified PDSA approach with APP PCPI.

part of the Model of the Clinical Practice of Emergency Medicine, for example

- *Clinical care processes*
- *Feedback from patients that relates to the clinical care given*
- *Outcomes of clinical care*
- *Access to care such as time for through-put, left without being seen, etc*

Group data and data collected through a national, regional, or local practice improvement program in which you participate is acceptable.

2. Compare the data to evidence-based guidelines. Evidence-based guidelines are based on published research subject to peer review. Only if such guidelines are not available, you may use guidelines set by expert consensus or comparable peer data. Guidelines set by expert consensus are published, accepted, national standards, and guidelines set by peer data are set by individuals who practice in like or similar circumstances.

   For measures for which there are no readily available benchmarks, the first measure set can be used as a baseline for future comparison. Nonetheless, there should be a clearly defined metric to monitor change in performance.

3. Develop and implement a plan to improve the practice issue measured in Step #1. You may plan for an individual or group improvement effort.

   Improvement interventions can be as simple as reporting results at a department meeting with suggestions for improvement, or as elaborate as a LEAN intervention (eg, a Kaizen event). *The key element is that the individual physician chooses to amend his or her behavior to improve performance.* Other forms of intervention could be a topic-specific journal club, monthly posting of data in the ED, or the development of condition-specific treatment guidelines (eg, instituting a pediatric asthma protocol).[5]

4. After implementing the improvement plan, review patient clinical care data from 10 additional patients with the same presentation, disease, or clinical process as the first patient data review. Use these data to evaluate whether clinical performance has been improved or maintained.

Note that the PCPI focus can be on individual care, *clinical care processes, outcomes of clinical care,* but can also be operational measures that affect all patients and physicians practicing within the department (Table 4a-2).

■ **TABLE 4A-2.** Options of APP PCPI Focus

Options of APP PCPI Focus	Example
1. Individual outcome	Successful pain control in digital block
2. Clinical care processes	CT utilization in renal colic
3. Operational measures	Time to provider, LOS in septic patients
4. ±Core measures	STEMI, PNA

In most cases, your data will (might) *be incorporated into department-wide initiatives. It is acceptable to use group data if that is the primary metric by which improvement is being measured. Still, individual performance data is typically the most effective information to assess your knowledge and skills.*[5]

The ABEM encourages physicians to use any local or national program, consider a clinical auditing program as in Chapter 3, or can develop a PCPI activity individually. Since all practicing emergency physicians have this MOC requirement, it makes great sense for the group to develop a strong clinical auditing program that meets every physician's requirement.

If the emergency department (ED) or your physician group is looking at patients with low-frequency, high-acuity conditions (such as acute myocardial infarction, stroke, or neutropenic fever), then fewer than ten patients is acceptable as long as some of your patients are included in the measurement group.[5]

The ABEM continues with describing "Acceptable Types of Patient Care Practice Improvement Activities." This list includes the established core measures of acute myocardial infarction and pneumonia as well as PQRS measures. While these are important clinical measures, the measures are less focused on individual physician decision making or application of knowledge base. Moreover, as observed at most facilities perhaps due to the hospital-based financial penalty involved in poor compliance, activity and completion of these measures have been standardized, almost automated, and now are largely outside of the individual physician decision making (for good or bad). Examples are aspirin on arrival for AMI (arguably not an ED measure as the requirement is within 24 hours of arrival), oxygenation assessment for pneumonia patients (should be automatic with VS and a nursing requirement), as well as sepsis and stroke protocols. Moreover, several examples are not pure EM requirements: ACE inhibitors given for LVSD and β-blocker within 24 hours of arrival.

The ABEM continues this pattern of including departmental performance measures in its "Case Studies in MOC" section.[5] The four cases described are core measures for CAP, door-to-balloon Six Sigma project, EKG-to-read times, and throughput times. Again, though these are worthy performance measures for a department, they do not represent individual practice and thus do not represent an individual's MOC and board certification status. For completion within a group practice, these measures may not have enough numbers of patients to meaningfully represent practice.

In conclusion, ABEM is blending a focus on an individual physician's practice quality with organizational or department goals. The opportunity to evoke a change in practice may not be easy though compliance with the requirement may be achieved if it is incorporated into a departmental focus. If you consider the topic of ASA with all STEMIs, most facilities have automated this to the point that the metric is nearly 100% compliant. Achieving any individually meaningful practice goals would be difficult as (1) the physician has limited control over the activity and (2) the opportunity for improvement is not great.

> **■ TABLE 4A-3.** Suggestions to Select a PCPI Topic
>
> 1. High frequency presentations
> 2. Intriguing topic in the literature that defines our specialty and in which you can visualize improvement
> 3. Care processes should impact your practice

Instead of the ABEM suggestions, I would like to propose an outline that would allow the physician to complete this activity and clinically benefit from the activity (Table 4a-3):

a. Choose a topic with high frequency of patients—you then have an opportunity to rapidly complete the activity.

   i. Ten patients with renal colic occur more frequently than 10 patients with Stevens-Johnson syndrome.

   ii. Ten patients in which the consideration of PE and assessment occur more frequently than 10 patients with the diagnosis of PE.

b. Choose a topic within the literature that encourages you to modify your practice.

   i. LLSA 2014 articles are probably better than 2004 articles.

   ii. Those topics that define our specialty (cardiopulmonary resuscitation, etc).

   iii. Keep it simple—ACEP has clinical policies that we all could be more consistent with.

c. If you chose a care process instead of a disease presentation, it should be a process that specifically impacts your practice and has meaning to you.

   i. How often do we review VS prior to discharging a patient? Can I use this activity to change my practice pattern according to this care process?

In the subsequent section I have developed some topics for the APP PCPI requirement. These are current as of this publication. The templates are individually focused and reviewed for your use.

■ DOES THE APP PCPI REQUIREMENT ADD TO TECHNICAL QUALITY?

It is this author's opinion that the ABEM APP PCPI requirement will be unable to raise and sustain an individual's comprehensive practice. Consider the current requirements:

- *Clinically active diplomates must begin, complete, and attest to completion of one PI activity in years one through five of their certification, and one PI activity in years six through ten.*

- *Review patient clinical care data from ten of your patients.*[4]

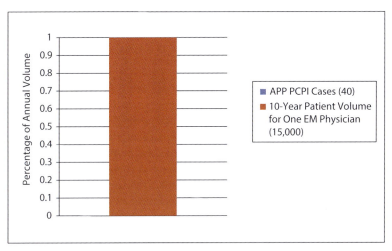

FIGURE 4A-3. Comparison of APP PCPI case volume to total practice volume (%)—one emergency physician.

Similar to the criticism of peer review (Chapter 2), APP PCPI poorly represents a comprehensive view of a physician's practice; both the frequency and the volume as required are inadequate as representation of a practice, for any significant practice monitoring or to show the incorporation of LLSA or ongoing medical learning. This is not a new complaint, and Brennan mentions sample size limitations as one of three challenges to including physician competence in health care quality.[6] If a group has no formal clinical review process, and the BCEM physician sees 1500-2500 patients annually, the APP PCPI process represents less than 0.1% of the patients managed over 5 years (Figure 4a-3). This again is inadequate representation of practice and would not show knowledge translation (incorporation of LLSA) or what aspects of a physician's practice have atrophied.

On a positive note, the APP PCPI requirement is sound in method as it encourages review of disease presentations, requires an EBM comparative platform, and invokes a method of improvement format that includes subsequent review of patients (Table 4a-4).

- *The data must be related to a single presentation, disease, or clinical care process that is part of the Model of the Clinical Practice of Emergency Medicine*
- *Compare the data to evidence-based guidelines*

■ TABLE 4A-4. Positive Components of APP PCPI Requirement and Methodology
1. Can include disease presentations
2. Requires comparison to EBM literature
3. Uses methods of improvement including pre- and postchange assessments

- *After implementing the improvement plan, review patient clinical care data from ten additional patients with the same presentation, disease, or clinical process as the first patient data review. Use this data to evaluate whether clinical performance has been improved or maintained.*[4]

And retrospectively, the evolution of ABEM's MOC is a pattern of increased frequency with the current requirements of approximately annual LLSA testing as well as the introduction of assessment (APP) every 5 years. This direction is consistent with increased intensity of high-value practice intervention produced within the SCA method and advocated for overall effective performance improvement.[7] Understandably, ABEM policy attempts to weigh cost and time commitments of its parties; despite the low frequency and small volumes, this requirement is a meaningful step to an advocate of intensive technical monitoring. The Sequential Clinical Auditing program as described in Chapter 3 would easily and efficiently provide the specificity and volume of patients for individual physicians to complete the APP PCPI requirement *and* be a method of raising and sustaining individual and group performance. In fact, having a comprehensive clinical auditing program would automate each individual physician's APP PCPI requirement and compliance within the group (Figure 4a-4).

As expected, the ACEP has also become involved with the APP requirement. In its web site advertisement it provides access to several topics on improving patient safety as part of completing the APP PCPI component.[8] The topics currently for sale are "Improving the Handoff Process" and "Planning Safer & More Effective Aftercare." Again, this product or service is not particularly focused on clinical accuracy or knowledge translation. The emphasis on patient safety may be coming from the ABMS 2014 standards which have a focus on patient safety.[9] Again, much of this is operational and does not assess clinical accuracy and diagnostic or technical outcomes.

■ ATTESTATION

The ABEM is fairly straightforward with the attestation requirement as there are three necessary components:
The physician must use the defined steps for the APP activity.

1. Review clinical care data from at least 10 of the physician's patients with the same clinical issue (fewer than 10 is acceptable for important clinical issues of lower prevalence and higher acuity).
2. Compare the data to evidence-based guidelines or other available benchmarks.
3. Implement a plan to improve the practice issue measured in Step #1.
4. After implementing the improvement plan, review patient clinical care data for the same clinical issue from an additional 10 of the physician's patients (again, fewer than 10 patients is acceptable for important high-acuity/low-volume clinical issues).

The ABEM will not accept any patient data (but states that 10% of activity will be "randomly selected for verification" so save your data!).

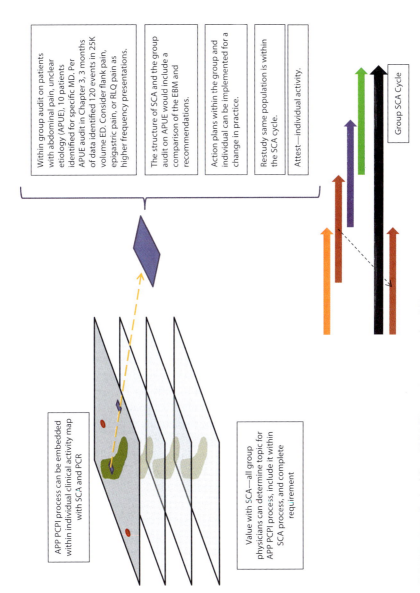

Within group audit on patients with abdominal pain, unclear etiology (APUE), 10 patients identified for specific MD. Per APUE audit in Chapter 3, 3 months of data identified 120 events in 25K volume ED. Consider flank pain, epigastric pain, or RLQ pain as higher frequency presentations.

The structure of SCA and the group audit on APUE would include a comparison of the EBM and recommendations.

Action plans within the group and individual can be implemented for a change in practice.

Restudy same population is within the SCA cycle.

Attest—individual activity.

Group SCA Cycle

APP PCPI process can be embedded within individual clinical activity map with SCA and PCR

Value with SCA—all group physicians can determine topic for APP PCPI process, include it within SCA process, and complete requirement

FIGURE 4A–4. Embedding APP PCPI requirement within SCA.

■ VERIFICATION OF ACTIVITY

The physician must identify another individual ("someone with oversight or knowledge of practice performance") who can verify the quality improvement activity (departmental chair, medical director, etc). See the ABEM Web site for electronic attestation and verification for your activity.

■ EXAMPLES FOR COMPLIANCE WITH THE APP PCPI COMPONENT

The following are nine templates board-certified emergency physicians could consider for use in order to complete the APP PCPI requirement. In considering source materials and selecting targets, it is reasonable to look to the literature within the LLSA yearly lists as well as reviewing the major EM journals for opportunities of practice change. Probably the most valued sources are the ACEP clinical policies as the APP PCPI requirement suggests guidelines should be primary foci or sources.

Considering the source of the project, the articles should be good, current EBM examples that would encourage the employing physician to a heightened level of practice. Included within the templates and according to the evoked EBM are proposed clinical goals for practice change. These are fairly straightforward but if the user disagrees with any part modify accordingly and reference the literature according to the position! As much as the ABEM proposes a group process and advocates for operational topics, this is an individual practice improvement effort; do what is necessary and efficient to support your own practice change.

Some may question the "here it is" approach provided in this text. In the author's mind the goal of the APP PCPI is not to teach anyone about setting up an audit or review but to potentiate a successful effort at modifying individual clinical practice for the better. It is also important to consider that confirming high-quality/consistent care with a guideline or a policy is a goal in itself.

Finding patients based on the topic may be challenging depending on your documentation system. Contact your coding person or business contact and request 20 patients according to the diagnosis and within a time period. The coder should be able to provide a list based on diagnosis code. Some patients are miscoded and thus the reason for 20 patients though you only need 10.

It should be easy to enter either the patient's name or the MRN into the EMR you are using, pull up the chart and abstract it. Similar methods can be used post-intervention to collect your comparative data. If you are still (strangely) on paper records, I assume you know where the medical records department is in your hospital!

And finally, in preparation of this text and specifically this chapter, the author submitted the template format to the ABEM for a determination on whether the textbook format complies with the ABEM criteria for externally developed APP activities. The ABEM's description of externally developed APP activities is largely instruction to corporations or organizations that plan to provide APP activities and CME as a business venture. In the author's mind, a textbook on practice performance is not consistent with the externally developed APP activities and the ABEM agreed: A textbook did not meet the criteria for an external APP program. This is due to (from the ABEM response letter):

(1) "Expert review and revision of the activity should occur at least once every three years" and that a textbook edition cycle may not be updated as frequently. These templates are an up-to-date framework on which an individual physician can organize an improvement topic. I recommend that the physician always review the ABEM Website for any changes to the ABEM requirement prior to using any suggested template in this section or any external program. The template format is directly from the ABEM Web site as if an individual was developing his or her own project. The ABEM only refers to the frequency of a publication but not the structure of the template.

(2) The ABEM describes the externally developed APP activity as one that should provide CME for participation. To this end, this textbook will not provide CME but provides a template to make completion of this requirement as feasible as possible without additional cost.

Adult Seizure Management

1. Guideline or Literature Associated with Topic: Clinical Policy: Critical Issues in the Evaluation and Management of Adult Patients Presenting to the Emergency Department With Seizures.[10] NOTE: PRIOR TO INITIATING THIS REVIEW A REVIEW OF THE CLINICAL POLICY AND ABEM'S APP PCPI POLICY IS REQUIRED—THIS FORM REPRESENTS A SIMPLIFIED WORK SHEET.

2. Goals:

   a. In patients with a first generalized convulsive seizure who have returned to their baseline clinical status:

      i. "Emergency physicians need not initiate antiepileptic medication* in the ED for patients who have had a first provoked seizure. Precipitating medical conditions should be identified and treated...Provoked/ causes: Seizures from hyponatremia or other electrolyte abnormalities, withdrawal, toxic ingestions, encephalitis, CNS mass lesions, etc. Unprovoked: epilepsy, distant stroke, distant TBI."

         1. *Reduce initiating long-term antiepileptic treatment in provoked seizures.*

            a. *Manage acute seizure activity as required.*

         2. *Consider admission in patients with first-time provoked seizures.*

      ii. "Emergency physicians need not initiate antiepileptic medication in the ED for patients who have had a first unprovoked seizure without evidence of brain disease or injury."

         1. *Reduce initiating long-term antiepileptic treatment in first-time unprovoked seizures.*

            a. *Manage acute seizure activity as required.*

         2. *Reduce hospitalization frequency in patients with first-time unprovoked seizure and normal mental status (return to baseline)*

      iii. "Emergency physicians may initiate antiepileptic medication in the ED, or defer in coordination with other providers, for patients who experienced a first unprovoked seizure with a remote history of brain disease or injury."

         1. *Consider initiating long-term antiepileptic treatment in first-time unprovoked seizures with history of TBI, CVA, etc.*

            a. *Manage acute seizure activity as required.*

         2. *Consider consulting or referral to neurology.*

   b. In patients with a known seizure disorder in which "resuming their antiepileptic medication in the ED is deemed appropriate... IV or oral medication" is allowed.

      i. *Increase or sustain frequency of restarting antiepileptic medication in ED patients with known seizure disorder.*

c. "In ED patients with generalized convulsive status epilepticus who continue to have seizures despite receiving optimal dosing of a benzodiazepine," several agents should be administered subsequently:

i. *Increase or sustain frequency of administration of intravenous phenytoin, fosphenytoin, or valproate (primary agents) in ED patients with refractory status epilepticus who have failed treatment with benzodiazepines.*

ii. *Consider secondary agents intravenous levetiracetam, propofol, or barbiturates in ED patients with refractory status epilepticus who have failed treatment with benzodiazepines.*

3. Data on First 10 Patients: Use Table 4a-5

4. Plan to Improve:
I have selected all or some of the goals as described. I have/have not amended those goals according to my site of practice, current literature, or due to another focus in clinical practice. These amendments are below.

In order to improve my care, I have:

a. ___ Amended my discharge instructions to incorporate the new knowledge

b. ___ Amended my chart documentation

c. ___ Made a presentation to my group confirming my knowledge of the literature on this topic

d. ___ Have developed a personal reminder to support my awareness of the topic while practicing

e. ___ Compiled and/or authored and/or championed a guideline for this topic within my institution

f. ___ Other:

5. Data on Second 10 Patients: Use Table 4a-5

6. Summary:

7. Attestation: *ABEM will not accept any patient data. See the Attestation section for directions on completing an attestation according to ABEM requirements. The physician must identify another individual ("someone with oversight or knowledge of practice performance") who can verify the quality improvement activity (departmental chair, medical director, etc).*

■ TABLE 4A-5. Adult Seizure Management—Pre- and Postdata

Patient #	Type: First Seizure—P	Type: First Seizure—U	Type: First Seizure—UI	NCCT Y/N	Start Long-Term A-E Rx (First Sz) Y/N	Admitted Y/N	Type: Known Sz Disorder; Return to Baseline?	Restart Long-Term A-E Rx (Known Sz) Y/N	Admitted Y/N	If Status Epilepticus, Agent of Choice
1										
2										
3										
4										
5										
6										
7										
8										
9										
10										

NCCT = noncontrast CT head.

Sz = seizure

First seizure: P = provoked; U = unprovoked (see text); UI = unprovoked + CNS injury hx

A-E Rx = antiepileptic treatment

Status meds: P = phenytoin; f = fosphenytoin; V = valproate; k = Keppra; PR = propofol; b = barbiturate

Seizure and Neuroimaging

It is interesting that the above 2014 ACEP clinical policy on seizures no longer includes a neuroimaging discussion. The authors address this gap: "The American College of Emergency Physicians' (ACEP) 2004 clinical policy on seizures addressed 2 critical questions on laboratory testing and neuroimaging: ... (2) Which new-onset seizure patients who have returned to a normal baseline require a head computed tomography (CT) scan in the ED? The committee agreed that these areas were no longer controversial and did not readdress these questions in the current draft."

Though the literature and the policy position have not changed for ACEP; it is apparent that with many physicians (providers) and in many EDs, head CT imaging for seizure patients is frequent and overused. Therefore, I have included an addendum with the current PI module for the ACEP seizure policy and encourage a utilization review on your practice and this topic. A review of the 2004 policy is below as well as a data form which could be included or separate from the prior seizure APP PCPI format.

1. Guideline or Literature Associated with Topic: Practice Parameter: Neuroimaging in the Emergency Patient Presenting With Seizure (Summary Statement).[11] NOTE: PRIOR TO INITIATING THIS REVIEW A REVIEW OF THE CLINICAL POLICY IS REQUIRED—THIS FORM REPRESENTS A SIMPLIFIED WORK SHEET.

2. Goals:
   Neuroimaging (NI) can help determine whether seizures result from a structural abnormality of the brain or its surroundings.

   a. *Increase or maintain frequency of ED imaging of first-time seizure patients.*

   b. *Decrease the frequency of ED imaging on patients with known seizure disorder, typical recurrent seizure, and normal neurological examination [return to baseline].*

      i. *Imaging should be performed when return to baseline status has not occurred or when structural lesion is suspected.*

3. Data on 10 Patients: See Table 4a-6

4. Continue as with ACEP Seizure Policy format

■ TABLE 4A-6.   Seizure and Neuroimaging—Pre- and Postdata

Patient #	New Onset + NCCT	Recurrent Sz + NCCT	Recurrent Sz Indications for Imaging							
			Indic: Concern for IC Process	Indic: CHI, Cancer, Immunocompromised	Indic: Fever (Meningitis + Focal Examination)	Indic: Persist HA	Indic: Anticoagulation	Indic: Focal CNS Examination	Indic: > 40 years	Indic: New Pattern
#1-10										

NCCT = noncontrast CT head
Sz = seizure
Indic = indication for imaging in recurrent seizure patient
IC = intracranial process
CHI = closed head injury
HA = headache
CNS = central nervous system

Adult Asymptomatic HTN Management

1. Guideline or Literature Associated with Topic: Clinical Policy: Critical Issues in the Evaluation and Management of Adult Patients in the Emergency Department With Asymptomatic Elevated Blood Pressure.[12] NOTE: PRIOR TO INITIATING THIS REVIEW A REVIEW OF THE CLINICAL POLICY AND ABEM'S APP PCPI POLICY IS REQUIRED—THIS FORM REPRESENTS A SIMPLIFIED WORK SHEET.

2. Goals:

   a. In ED patients with asymptomatic elevated blood pressure, screening for target organ injury does not reduce rates of adverse outcomes. "Routine screening for acute target organ injury (eg, serum creatinine, urinalysis, ECG) is not required. In select patient populations (eg, poor follow-up), screening for an elevated serum creatinine level may identify kidney injury that affects disposition (eg, hospital admission)."

      i. *Decrease frequency of screening tests for end-organ injury in patients with asymptomatic hypertension.*

   b. "In patients with asymptomatic markedly elevated blood pressure, ED medical intervention is not required. In select patient populations (eg, poor follow-up), emergency physicians may treat markedly elevated blood pressure in the ED and/or initiate therapy for long-term control. [Consensus recommendation] and should be referred for outpatient follow-up. [Consensus recommendation]"

      i. *Decrease the frequency of medical intervention for asymptomatic HTN in the ED*

      ii. *Option B: Initiate therapy for long-term control for asymptomatic HTN in the ED*

      iii. *Option C: Initiate more consistent or specific outpatient follow-up.*

3. Data on First 10 Patients: See Table 4a-7.

4. Plan to Improve:
   I have selected all or some of the goals as described. I have/have not amended those goals according to my site of practice, current literature, or due to another focus in clinical practice. These amendments are below.

   In order to improve my care, I have:

   a. ___ Amended my discharge instructions to incorporate the new knowledge

   b. ___ Amended my chart documentation

   c. ___ Made a presentation to my group confirming my knowledge of the literature on this topic

   d. ___ Have developed a personal reminder to support my awareness of the topic while practicing

   e. ___ Compiled and/or authored and/or championed a guideline for this topic within my institution

   f. ___ Other:

Patient #	ED Screening Tests (Cr, UA, ECG) Y/N	Decision to Rx in the ED Y/N	Start (Restart) Outpatient Rx Y/N	Notation of Specific Follow-up Plan With PCP, Access to Rx/Meds
#1-10				

■ **TABLE 4A-7.** Adult Asymptomatic HTN Management—Pre- and Postdata

Cr = serum creatinine; UA = urinalysis; ECG = electrocardiogram
Rx = medication treatment
PCP = primary care provider

5. Data on Second 10 Patients: See Table 4a-7.

6. Summary:

7. Attestation: *ABEM will not accept any patient data. See the Attestation section for directions on completing an attestation according to ABEM requirements. The physician must identify another individual ("someone with oversight or knowledge of practice performance") who can verify the quality improvement activity (departmental chair, medical director, etc).*

Early Pregnancy

1. Guideline or Literature Associated with Topic: Clinical Policy: Critical Issues in the Initial Evaluation and Management of Patients Presenting to the Emergency Department in Early Pregnancy[13] and Ectopic Pregnancy.[14] NOTE: PRIOR TO INITIATING THIS REVIEW A REVIEW OF THE CLINICAL POLICY AND ABEM'S APP PCPI POLICY IS REQUIRED—THIS FORM REPRESENTS A SIMPLIFIED WORK SHEET.

2. Goals:

    a. Per the guideline: "…It is well documented that ectopic pregnancies can present at almost any hCG level, high or low. Some clinicians may defer an ultrasound when the hCG level is below the discriminatory threshold because they think that the risk of rupture is low. However, rupture has been documented at very low hCG levels."

       i. *Increase or maintain the frequency of obtaining a pelvic ultrasound for symptomatic pregnant patients with an hCG level at any discriminatory threshold.*

          1. *Do not use the hCG value to exclude the diagnosis of ectopic pregnancy in patients who have an indeterminate ultrasound.*

       ii. *Increase or maintain the frequency of specialty consultation or arrangement of close outpatient follow-up for all patients with an indeterminate pelvic ultrasound.*

    b. In patients receiving methotrexate for confirmed or suspected ectopic pregnancy:

       i. *Increase or maintain the frequency of outpatient follow-up for patients who receive MTX therapy in the ED for a confirmed or suspected EP.*

          1. *Strongly consider ruptured ectopic pregnancy in the differential diagnosis of patients who have received MTX and present with concerning signs or symptoms.*

    c. In patients with threatened abortion, complete abortion, ectopic pregnancy, and minor abdominal trauma:

       i. *Increase or maintain the frequency of administering 50 μg of Rhogam to Rh-negative women in all cases of documented first-trimester loss of established pregnancy.*

3. Data on First 10 Patients: Table 4a-8

4. Plan to Improve:

    I have selected all or some of the goals as described. I have/have not amended those goals according to my site of practice, current literature, or due to another focus in clinical practice. These amendments are below.

    In order to improve my care, I have:

    a. ____ Amended my discharge instructions to incorporate the new knowledge

    b. ____ Amended my chart documentation

    c. ____ Made a presentation to my group confirming my knowledge of the literature on this topic

■ **TABLE 4A-8.** Symptomatic[a] Early Pregnancy—Pre- and Post-data

Patient #	hCG	US	If Indeterminate Status After US, Document OB Referral in 2 days	Rhogam if indicated[b]	If MTX, Document OB Follow- Up Plan
#1-10					

[a]Symptomatic = abdominal pain; vaginal bleeding and + qualitative hCG
hCG = quantitative hCG (level)
US =pelvic ultrasound
OB =obstetrical
[b]Indications: threatened Ab; complete Ab; ectopic pregnancy; minor abdominal trauma
MTX = methotrexate

    d. ___ Have developed a personal reminder to support my awareness of the topic while practicing

    e. ___ Compiled and/or authored and/or championed a guideline for this topic within my institution

    f. ___ Other:

5. <u>Data on Second 10 Patients</u>: Table 4a-8.

6. <u>Summary</u>:

7. <u>Attestation</u>: *ABEM will not accept any patient data. See the Attestation section for directions on completing an attestation according to ABEM requirements. The physician must identify another individual ("someone with oversight or knowledge of practice performance") who can verify the quality improvement activity (departmental chair, medical director, etc).*

Suspected Pulmonary Embolism

1. <u>Guideline or Literature Associated with Topic</u>: Critical Issues in the Evaluation and Management of Adult Patients Presenting to the Emergency Department With Suspected Pulmonary Embolism.[15] NOTE: PRIOR TO INITIATING THIS REVIEW A REVIEW OF THE CLINICAL POLICY AND ABEM'S APP PCPI POLICY IS REQUIRED – THIS FORM REPRESENTS A SIMPLIFIED WORK SHEET.

2. <u>Goals</u>:
   a. Either objective criteria or gestalt clinical assessment can be used to risk stratify patients with suspected PE. There is insufficient evidence to support the preferential use of one method over another.
      i. *Increase the frequency of documenting clinical decision rules (confirm use) or use of gestalt in considering PE as etiology of patient symptom, OR*
      ii. *Increase frequency of using the PERC to exclude the diagnosis based on historical and physical examination data alone (reducing testing), OR*
      iii. *Increase frequency of using a negative quantitative D-dimer assay result to exclude PE in patients with low pretest probability for PE.*
   b. CT pulmonary angiogram as the sole diagnostic test in the exclusion of PE:
      i. *Increase the frequency of use of CT pulmonary angiogram to exclude PE when the patient is low risk per clinical decision rule but with a positive D-dimer assay*
   c. Venous ultrasound as a diagnostic test in the exclusion of PE:
      i. *Increase the frequency of use of DVT studies to exclude VTE when the patient is moderate/intermediate to high risk per clinical decision rule and CT pulmonary angiogram is negative for PE.*
      ii. *Consider venous ultrasound to confirm DVT in patients with PE symptoms to reduce further imaging and to initiate treatment.*
   d. Thrombolytic treatment in patients with PE:
      i. *Increase the frequency of thrombolytic therapy in hemodynamically unstable patients with confirmed PE for whom the benefits of treatment outweigh the risks of life-threatening bleeding complications.*

3. <u>Data on First 10 Patients</u>: Table 4a-9

4. <u>Plan to Improve</u>:
   I have selected all or some of the goals as described. I have/have not amended those goals according to my site of practice, current literature, or due to another focus in clinical practice. These amendments are below.

   In order to improve my care, I have:
   a. ___ Amended my discharge instructions to incorporate the new knowledge
   b. ___ Amended my chart documentation
   c. ___ Made a presentation to my group confirming my knowledge of the literature on this topic

■ **TABLE 4A-9.** Symptoms c/w Suspected Pulmonary Embolism Pre- and Post-data

Patient #	PERC to Exclude PE	Wells Exclusion: Low Prob. + Low D-Dimer	Other Clinical Decision Tool to Exclude	Wells: CT Pulmonary Angiography If Low Prob. + High D-Dimer	Venous US for DVT If Wells Mod to High Risk + Neg. CT Pulmonary Angiography	Consider Thrombolytics in Unstable Pts With Confirmed PE
#1-10						

PERC = pulmonary embolism (PE) rule-out criteria
Wells = Wells criteria
Prob. = probability
US = ultrasound
DVT = deep venous thrombosis

    d. ___ Have developed a personal reminder to support my awareness of the topic while practicing

    e. ___ Compiled and/or authored and/or championed a guideline for this topic within my institution

    f. ___ Other:

5. Data on Second 10 Patients: Table 4a-9

6. Summary:

7. Attestation: *ABEM will not accept any patient data. See the Attestation section for directions on completing an attestation according to ABEM requirements. The physician must identify another individual ("someone with oversight or knowledge of practice performance") who can verify the quality improvement activity (departmental chair, medical director, etc).*

Acute Abdominal Pain, Risk of Appendicitis

1. Guideline or Literature Associated with Topic: Clinical Policy: Critical Issues in the Evaluation and Management of Emergency Department Patients With Suspected Appendicitis.[16] NOTE: PRIOR TO INITIATING THIS REVIEW A REVIEW OF THE CLINICAL POLICY AND ABEM'S APP PCPI POLICY IS REQUIRED – THIS FORM REPRESENTS A SIMPLIFIED WORK SHEET.

2. Goals:

   a. "In patients with suspected acute appendicitis, use clinical findings (ie, signs and symptoms) to risk-stratify patients and guide decisions about further testing (eg, no further testing, laboratory tests, and/or imaging studies), and management (eg, discharge, observation, and/or surgical consultation)."

      i. *Increase the use of specific history and physical examination in considering the potential for appendicitis.*

      ii. *Increase the frequency of use of EB components in appendicitis in determining further evaluation and disposition.*

         1. *Consider using the Alvarado score in the assessment of patients for appendicitis.*

   b. "In adult patients undergoing a CT scan for suspected appendicitis, perform abdominal and pelvic CT scan with or without contrast (intravenous [IV], oral, or rectal). The addition of IV and oral contrast may increase the sensitivity of the CT scan for the diagnosis of appendicitis." Author's note: Currently use of NCCT is more standard in EM.[17]

      i. *Increase the frequency of noncontrast or IV-only contrast abdominal-pelvic CT scans for the diagnosis of appendicitis.*

   c. "In children, use ultrasound to confirm acute appendicitis but not to definitively exclude acute appendicitis…Given the concern over exposing children to ionizing radiation, consider using ultrasound as the initial imaging modality. In cases in which the diagnosis remains uncertain after ultrasound, CT may be performed."

      i. *Increase or maintain the use of US as the initial imaging choice for children with suspected appendicitis.*

   d. Pain treatment prior to completing full examination will improve patient satisfaction and potentially improve the clinical evaluation.[18]

      i. *Increase the frequency of pain medication administration early in the abdominal pain evaluation.*

   e. Appropriate disposition and request for return or reevaluation.

      i. *Increase or maintain the advocacy of return and reevaluation within 2 days.*

    f. Literature identifies these patients, age >55 and/or with vascular or immunocompromising diseases, when presenting with APUE, as having significantly increased morbidity and mortality.[19] It is advocated that these patients should return to the ED, considering the high frequency of admission, risk of pathology, and accessibility to further imaging studies, testing and consultation.

        i. *Maintain and/or increase the comprehensive examinations in all high-risk patients.*

        ii. *Increase recommendation for reevaluation in <2 days, especially in all high-risk patients.*

3. <u>Data on First 10 Patients</u>: Table 4a-10

4. <u>Plan to Improve</u>:

I have selected all or some of the goals as described. I have/have not amended those goals according to my site of practice, current literature, or due to another focus in clinical practice. These amendments are below.

In order to improve my care, I have:

a. ___ Amended my discharge instructions to incorporate the new knowledge

b. ___ Amended my chart documentation

c. ___ Made a presentation to my group confirming my knowledge of the literature on this topic

d. ___ Have developed a personal reminder to support my awareness of the topic while practicing

e. ___ Compiled and/or authored and/or championed a guideline for this topic within my institution

f. ___ Other:

5. <u>Data on Second 10 Patients</u>: Table 4a-10

■ TABLE 4A-10. Acute Abdominal Pain, Risk of Appendicitis—Pre- and Postdata

Patient #	High Risk Patient?	Pain Medication	In Adult Patients, NC or IV Contrast Only A/P CT	In Pediatric Patients, US First	If Discharged, Recommend Follow-Up in 1-2 Days
#1-10					

High risk = > 55 years old and /or vascular or immunocompromised disease – approach: increase comprehensive examination
NC = noncontrast
A/P CT = abdominal/pelvic computerized tomography
US = ultrasound

6. Summary:

7. Attestation: *ABEM will not accept any patient data. See the Attestation section for directions on completing an attestation according to ABEM requirements. The physician must identify another individual ("someone with oversight or knowledge of practice performance") who can verify the quality improvement activity (departmental chair, medical director, etc).*

Acute Headache

1. <u>Guideline or Literature Associated with Topic</u>: Clinical Policy: Critical Issues in the Evaluation and Management of Adult Patients Presenting to the Emergency Department With Acute Headache.[20] NOTE: PRIOR TO INITIATING THIS REVIEW A REVIEW OF THE CLINICAL POLICY AND ABEM'S APP PCPI POLICY IS REQUIRED – THIS FORM REPRESENTS A SIMPLIFIED WORK SHEET.

2. <u>Goals</u>: "Emergency physicians must determine which patients need neuroimaging in the ED and which can be appropriately deferred and evaluated in the outpatient setting. Many patients have limited access to care, which further complicates this decision process in clinical practice."

   a. Patients present to the ED for pain control, several guidelines encourage the use of nonnarcotic management:

      i. *Decrease the frequency of narcotic medications to control headaches.*

   b. The ED physician should consider the necessity of neuroimaging in all patients presenting with acute HA. "Patients presenting to the ED with headache and new abnormal findings in a neurologic examination (eg, focal deficit, altered mental status, altered cognitive function) should undergo emergent* noncontrast head CT. Patients presenting with new sudden-onset severe headache should undergo an emergent* head CT. HIV-positive patients with a new type of headache should be considered for an emergent* neuroimaging study. Patients who are older than 50 years and presenting with new type of headache but with a normal neurologic examination should be considered for an urgent† neuroimaging study."

      i. *Increase or maintain the frequency of NCCT for patients with new sudden-onset HA, with or without focal neuro deficits.*

      ii. *Increase or maintain the frequency of NCCT in all HIV+ patients with new HA.*

      iii. *Increase or maintain the frequency of NCCT in all patients with new-onset HA and >50 years old.*

      iv. *Reduce the frequency of NCCT for patients with recurrent, chronic HA.*

   c. "In patients presenting to the ED with sudden-onset, severe headache and a negative noncontrast head CT scan result, lumbar puncture should be performed to rule out subarachnoid hemorrhage." Controversy exists on the approach to further evaluating for SAH after a negative NCCT due to the increasing sensitivity of NCCT as well as the challenges of performing an LP[21-23] "Patients with a sudden-onset, severe headache who have negative findings on a head CT, normal opening pressure, and negative findings in CSF analysis do not need emergent angiography and can be discharged from the ED with follow-up recommended."

      i. *Increase the frequency of LP procedure to evaluate for SAH in ED patients with acute HA* <u>AND/OR</u>

ii. *Increase the frequency of IV-contrast CT or MR to evaluate for SAH in ED patients with acute HA.*

d. "Adult patients with headache and exhibiting signs of increased intracranial pressure (eg, papilledema, absent venous pulsations on funduscopic examination, altered mental status, focal neurologic deficits, signs of meningeal irritation) should undergo a neuroimaging study before having a lumbar puncture. In the absence of clinical findings suggestive of increased intracranial pressure, a lumbar puncture can be performed without obtaining a neuroimaging study. (Note: A lumbar puncture does not assess for all causes of a sudden severe headache.)"

i. *Decrease the frequency of NCCT when patients have no clinical findings of increased ICP prior to performing an LP.*

3. Data on First 10 Patients: Table 4a-11

4. Plan to Improve:

I have selected all or some of the goals as described. I have/have not amended those goals according to my site of practice, current literature, or due to another focus in clinical practice. These amendments are below.

In order to improve my care, I have:

a. ___ Amended my discharge instructions to incorporate the new knowledge

b. ___ Amended my chart documentation

c. ___ Made a presentation to my group confirming my knowledge of the literature on this topic

d. ___ Have developed a personal reminder to support my awareness of the topic while practicing

e. ___ Compiled and/or authored and/or championed a guideline for this topic within my institution

f. ___ Other:

■ **TABLE 4A-11.** Acute Headache—Pre- and Postdata

Patient #	Acute or Different HA Pattern[a]	Chronic, Recurrent HA	Non-narcotic Medication	NCCT	LP for SAH	CTA/ MR for SAH	NCCT pre-LP[b]
#1-10							

HA = headache
[a]High risk = new, different, HIV + history, or >50 years old with onset
NCCT = noncontrast computerized tomography
LP = lumbar puncture
SAH = subarachnoid hemorrhage
CTA = CT angiography
MR = magnetic resonance
[b]Focal examination or increased ICP

5. <u>Data on Second 10 Patients:</u> Table 4a-11

6. <u>Summary:</u>

7. <u>Attestation:</u> *ABEM will not accept any patient data. See the Attestation section for directions on completing an attestation according to ABEM requirements. The physician must identify another individual ("someone with oversight or knowledge of practice performance") who can verify the quality improvement activity (departmental chair, medical director, etc).*

Syncope

1. Guideline or Literature Associated with Topic: Clinical Policy: Critical Issues in the Evaluation and Management of Adult Patients Presenting to the Emergency Department with Syncope[24] and "Electrocardiogram Findings in Emergency Department Patients with Syncope."[25] NOTE: PRIOR TO INITIATING THIS REVIEW A REVIEW OF THE CLINICAL POLICY AND ABEM'S APP PCPI POLICY IS REQUIRED – THIS FORM REPRESENTS A SIMPLIFIED WORK SHEET.

2. Goals: "The traditional approach of focusing on establishing an etiology of syncope in the ED is often of limited utility. Multiple studies have demonstrated a diagnostic rate of only 20% to 50% in the initial evaluation of the syncope patient… Consider older age, structural heart disease, or a history of coronary artery disease as risk factors for adverse outcome. Consider younger patients with syncope that is nonexertional, without history or signs of cardiovascular disease, a family history of sudden death, and without comorbidities to be at low risk of adverse events."

    a. *Decrease the frequency of additional studies in patients with syncope with low risk of adverse events.*

    b. *Increase or maintain frequency on obtaining ECG in patients with syncope.*

    c. *Increase the frequency of documenting an indication for additional studies as related to possible increased risk of adverse events.*

    d. *Increase or maintain the frequency of admissions of patients with syncope and evidence of heart failure or structural heart disease.*

        i. *Increase or maintain the frequency of admission of patients with syncope and other factors that lead to stratification as high risk for adverse outcome : older age and associated comorbidities, abnormal ECG, Hct <30 (if obtained), history or presence of heart failure, coronary artery disease, or structural heart disease.*

3. Data on First 10 Patients: Table 4a-12

4. Plan to Improve:
    I have selected all or some of the goals as described. I have/have not amended those goals according to my site of practice, current literature, or due to another focus in clinical practice. These amendments are below.

    In order to improve my care, I have:

    a. ___ Amended my discharge instructions to incorporate the new knowledge

    b. ___ Amended my chart documentation

    c. ___ Made a presentation to my group confirming my knowledge of the literature on this topic

    d. ___ Have developed a personal reminder to support my awareness of the topic while practicing

    e. ___ Compiled and/or authored and/or championed a guideline for this topic within my institution

    f. ___ Other:

| ■ **TABLE 4A-12.** Syncope—Pre- and Postdata |

Patient #	Age[a]	Risk Factors Noted	Obtain ECG	Indications Noted for Extended Evaluation[b]	Admit
#1-10					

[a]Age > 65 years old = increased risk
Risk factors: age, abnormal ECG; lack of prodrome; Hx of CVD; Hx of CHF; SOB symptoms; hypotension on arrival; hct < 30.
[b]NC CT of head; CTA for PE; ECHO for aortic stenosis; CMP for severe hypokalemia, etc.

5. Data on Second 10 Patients: Table 4a-12

6. Summary:

7. Attestation: *ABEM will not accept any patient data. See the Attestation section for directions on completing an attestation according to ABEM requirements. The physician must identify another individual ("someone with oversight or knowledge of practice performance") who can verify the quality improvement activity (departmental chair, medical director, etc).*

Renal Colic

1. Guideline or Literature Associated with Topic: A Systematic Review of Medical Therapy to Facilitate Passage of Ureteral Calculi;[26] Association of Pyuria and Clinical Characteristics With the Presence of Urinary Tract Infection Among Patients With Acute Nephrolithiasis;[27] Acute Renal Colic from Ureteral Calculus;[28] ACR Appropriateness Criteria.[29] NOTE: PRIOR TO INITIATING THIS REVIEW A REVIEW OF THE CLINICAL POLICY AND ABEM'S APP PCPI POLICY IS REQUIRED – THIS FORM REPRESENTS A SIMPLIFIED WORK SHEET.

2. Goals:
   a. *Increase or maintain the frequency of obtaining urine for assessment of pregnancy and urinary tract infection.*
      i. *Consider necessity of obtaining UA in male with renal colic.[30]*
   b. *Consider nonnarcotic medications as initial treatment for suspected renal colic.*
   c. *Consider abdominal/pelvis NCCT in patients presenting with new flank pain and no history of renal colic.*
      i. *Consider renal US in all female patients with reproductive potential.*
   d. *Consider abdominal/pelvis NCCT or renal US in patients presenting with atypical or different symptoms of flank pain but with a history of renal colic.*
      i. *Consider renal US in all female patients with reproductive potential.*
      ii. *Consider evaluating renal function.*
   e. *Consider renal US in patients presenting with chronic flank pain and more than one NCCT of the abdomen and pelvis.*
      i. *Consider evaluating renal function.*
   f. *Increase frequency of prescribing "medical expulsive therapy," either α-antagonists or calcium channel blockers, to augment stone expulsion of distal ureteral stones.[26]*

3. Data on First 10 Patients: Table 4a-13

4. Plan to Improve:
   I have selected all or some of the goals as described. I have/have not amended those goals according to my site of practice, current literature, or due to another focus in clinical practice. These amendments are below.

   In order to improve my care, I have:
   a. ____ Amended my discharge instructions to incorporate the new knowledge
   b. ____ Amended my chart documentation
   c. ____ Made a presentation to my group confirming my knowledge of the literature on this topic
   d. ____ Have developed a personal reminder to support my awareness of the topic while practicing
   e. ____ Compiled and/or authored and/or championed a guideline for this topic within my institution
   f. ____ Other:

■ TABLE 4A-13. Renal Colic—Pre- and Post-data

Patient #	Initial Presentation	Recurrent Flank Pain*	Urinalysis With Pregnancy Test If Female	Non-narcotic Pain Medications as Initial Rx	NC A/P CT	Renal US	Medical Expulsive Rx on Discharge[b]
#1-10							

[a]Recurrent flank pain—consider serum Cr
Rx = treatment
NC A/P CT = noncontrast abdominal/pelvic computerized tomography
US = ultrasound
[b]α-antagonists and/or calcium-channel blockers

5. Data on Second 10 Patients: Table 4a-13

6. Summary:

7. Attestation: *ABEM will not accept any patient data. See the Attestation section for directions on completing an attestation according to ABEM requirements. The physician must identify another individual ("someone with oversight or knowledge of practice performance") who can verify the quality improvement activity (departmental chair, medical director, etc).*

Assessment of Practice Performance

4B: The ABEM APP Communication/ Professionalism Requirement

- **INTRODUCTION**
- **WHAT IS APP?**
- **ATTESTATION**

■ INTRODUCTION

I had a debate in my mind about including this topic in the textbook. This book's title, Assessment of Practice Performance in Emergency Medicine, can be inclusive of the ABEM's Communication/Professionalism requirement yet does not directly infer a discussion about patient satisfaction. The reader may, reacting to the excessive levels of patient satisfaction metrics and commentary in the trade journals, be cautious with my position. He or she may criticize this stance as a fine line; after all, the author promoted using aspects of hard quality to differentiate the group or organization within the market. Still, it is no trap; the author may innocently, indirectly teach you how to be a better salesperson but this was not his goal and he is doing his best to avoid it.

The patient satisfaction literature is weakly associated with clinical outcomes.[31] It leaves many confused; others take a side. An excessive patient satisfaction focus for financial gain is disingenuous and unprofessional; balance is needed. Organizations that overemphasize this are often forcing the physician into compromised decision making: complying with short term demands and satisfaction goals that have long-term consequences triggering negative health outcomes. All emergency physicians have seen patients presenting with *C difficile* colitis due to the excessive antibiotic provision in the community. The short-term gain of giving the antibiotic and pleasing the patient has put the patient at risk.[32,33]

We have seen that this focus can cause injury.[34] That is inexcusable. It would be acceptable if weak positive evidence was present without any negative study, but the moment any policy, much like drug studies, has a potential to harm, then it must be questioned or delayed, until better, safer therapy can be promoted. Yet, the indoctrinated continue to promote patient satisfaction with an odd logical linkage akin to a type I error.[35]

The difficulty physicians have with patient satisfaction and the business focus on this goal is fundamental. Arrow explored medical care as an object of normative economics and noted several conflicts of medical care with the competitive model.[36] First, there is unpredictable demand in which medical care provides satisfaction only in the departure from normal health. This can be observed in the emergency setting when the patient could be near death and is outside of rational decision making (presumed consent). Second, there is an imbalance of information related to skilled care such that the patient is unable to test the treatment before use. Since there is limited recourse in this one-directional exchange, the patient is reliant on trust in the brand. The appendix cannot be reintroduced and the patient shop for another surgeon to remove it again. You cannot test drive a hip replacement. This again addresses the challenge of the patient assessing the technical nature of medicine. It also makes it imperative that the physician emphasize accuracy as there could be no chance at clinical recovery compared to the known service recovery within normal business exchange. Third, and most pertinent to this discussion, is the necessity of objectivity of physicians. The concept of professionalism supports activity without promotion of self-interest; the physician is an expert in diagnosing and treating illness with an overall *concern for correctness*. The necessity of saying "no" or selectively providing limited care or even providing bad news that, however artfully delivered, will be less than satisfying and/or emotionally negative moves this service outside normative business exchange. This approach becomes difficult when the organization's self-interest is focused on maximizing the revenue from patient intervention and return patients conflicting with physician correctness and technical goals.

Referring back to the Bowers article introduced in the first chapter, it is clear that the authors of the paper defined the elements of technical quality apart from service quality.[37] Similarly, Sequist et al call for a separation as they found no significant correlation between patient experiences and clinical outcomes.[38] In simple analogy, two examples of this separation can be used from other businesses. First, computer programmers are the core technicians of most computer businesses and rarely are they involved with marketing the product. Instead, they are focused on the function and structure of the machine or software. Secondly, in Major League Baseball it is rare that the fourth or fifth batters in the lineup, those that often hit more homeruns and produce more RBIs, are given the signal to bunt. Their technical role on the team, evidenced by the lineup position even by the structure of their bodies, is to hit the homerun, not to bunt. Similarly in health care, it is important for roles to be maximized and for managers and leaders to link positions and roles into a highly functional team for patient betterment. Hospitals and health systems should promote individuals with service qualities who can align with a physician's technical work to achieve the duality of health and satisfaction. This is not discounting the need for communication and professionalism methods as this chapter will emphasize but it is trying to frame the discussion within organizations.

Perhaps in order to push their organizational goals some authors and leaders overextend the weak patient satisfaction literature aligned with the business side of health care to encompass clinical outcomes. They should be kept separate based on the above commentary, understanding that physicians personally want patients to be satisfied with their interaction, but we cannot step over the line and infer that a handshake and a smile will cure an illness. We cannot accept Moliere's opinion of medicine.

I would like to maintain the hard quality focus in this text when discussing the ABEM MOC APP Communication/Professionalism requirement, emphasizing the technical aspects of clinical care and linking some of the components promoted for patient satisfaction as valuable for clinical success. *Several activities noted in practicing medicine that raise patient satisfaction are legitimate aspects of technical practice.* In fact, focusing on these aspects of technical care could raise clinical quality, achieving health and satisfaction, the latter without directly focusing on it.

When we review the patient satisfaction literature, several outcomes associated with attempts to satisfy patients are described and these range from clinical goals to business goals. The three main clinical goals are diagnostic accuracy, symptom and problem resolution, and adherence to treatment plan (Figure 4b-1). The business goals are return clients for income generation (changing providers is a nonissue in emergency medicine with the exception of patients changing facilities [a multifactorial problem]), reduction in staff turnover for cost control (though

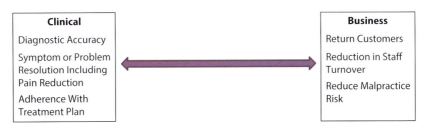

FIGURE 4B-1. Patient satisfaction dichotomy—clinical and business.

there would be an indirect value of a more efficient operations with less employee turnover as well as the association of employee satisfaction with customer satisfaction), and a reduced malpractice risk. Many could question the placement of malpractice events under the business heading. My reasons are such: First, there appears no predictability in the association of clinical outcomes to a lawsuit and there is a like-ability association. Second, the impact of a verdict in favor of the patient is often an exchange of money rather than a limiting of the practice of the physician (this may be due to a lack of physician oversight as well).

If we consider the evaluative process between the physician and the patient, the interview is frequently prior to the decision making and action (therapy). In emergency medicine it is the rare case, in critical care, in which the history and intervention is concurrent and thus we can say that most patients receive the sequence of history then physical examination prior to medical decision making and actions for therapy. The interview, a conversation between the physician and the patient, is the foremost step in diagnostic accuracy and successful clinical outcomes. Regardless of the satisfaction the patient receives in speaking about his or her problems and in being heard, the main focus of this step for the physician is obtaining data. Studies have shown that 70% to 80% of diagnoses are obtained through the history.[39,40] The data also show that the physical examination (12%) and subsequent testing (11%) do not recover accuracy but usually only supplement or reinforce the findings in the history[39] (Figure 4b-2). Thus, the irony described in Chapter 3 of some departments trying to do everything to everyone with a reliance on testing directly conflicts with the data that listening and asking questions rather than performing tests both heightens clinical accuracy, safety, and patient well-being. The linkage in this process to clinical outcomes is well envisioned. Obtaining early data that increase the probability of a diagnosis which is then confirmed or the likelihood further raised with an examination or testing is a strong step toward initiating proper treatment and thus leveraging the potential for expected outcomes (return to health, etc).

Extending this focus on the history of the chief complaint further, studies have shown that the uninterrupted chief complaint lasts on average 30 seconds.[41,42] If the goal was data extraction that could lead to a highly accurate diagnosis and successful treatment, physicians unfortunately show a pattern of interrupting patients prior to completion of their presenting complaint.[41] In this study, over 70% of patients were interrupted (or redirected) prior to their finishing their concerns which on average took only six more seconds to complete. Marvel et al showed that once the physician had interrupted the patient, the description of the issue was rarely completed (8%) (Figure 4b-3). In a study including emergency medicine residents, patients were interrupted within an average of 12 seconds after commencing a history and only

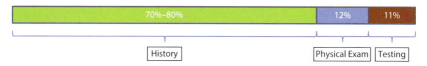

FIGURE 4B-2. Components of evaluative process resulting in diagnosis.

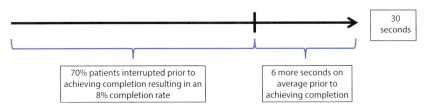

FIGURE 4B-3. Time and interruption description during chief complaint (not to scale).

20% concluded a history without interruption.[43] This is difficult. The concept that most physicians know that the history provides the most information to help the patient yet the pattern is one of interruption with loss of these valued data (presumably for efficiency) should lead us to review our practice approach and dedicate a new effort to listening if we are to technically maximize patient care.

Marvel further comments on the operational impact of interruptions: "multiple solicitations (open-ended questions) early in the visit may enhance the efficiency of the interview…allowing…the best use of their time" as they found that late-arising concerns occurred more frequently when the patients were interrupted (redirected). The data conflict with our general concept in which interruptions and focusing the patient result in a more efficient care event. It turns out we are often compromising efficiency.

Simply juxtaposing activities that could satisfy a patient, interruptions in comparison to allowing speech are unfavorable. Allowing the patient to speak without redirection can be a dual win of gaining more depth and accurate information of the presenting condition while affirming a patient's desire to communicate.

I will provide another comment on some emergency departments and the operational approach of the triage evaluation. Many emergency departments place MLPs into the triage arena to initiate care. It is doubtful due to the time and volume pressure in this area and contrasted with the RN triage method of simple, directed questions for bed placement and workload expectations that the MLP is allowing adequate time for the patient to express concerns without "redirecting." This activity is unfortunately procedurally constructed to compromise the retrieval of valuable, clinically directional data, and the result (observed by the author) is that procedures or testing are misused, overused, or even underused such that the "downstream" physician has often to add testing causing further delay (as noted in Marvel's article) or subtract and apologize for wasted time, testing, or painful unnecessary procedures. Again, this is a conflict of goals with a time to provider metric trumping efficient technical care but ultimately potentially causing a prolonged ED stay to "get it right."

The two subsequent clinical outcomes associated with patient satisfaction are symptom and/or problem resolution and the adherence to treatment plan relates more to actions within the emergency department stay as well as communication technique during and on discharge.

It is necessary to state the obvious: A physician's role is to manage a pathological process to relieve symptoms. The precise technical management of fixing what is not working or broken within the human body, of splinting a fracture or a digital block of a finger injury and the treatment of bronchospasm or nausea, is the work of physicians *and* satisfiers (it is satisfying to breathe). Sun et al found that more treatments within the department increased satisfaction.[32] Though this was a group with selected presentations (chest pain, asthma, etc) the treatments were not just focused on pain control. It cannot be surprising that patients enter the department expecting improvement, and providing the treatment with highest potential of success (scientifically based, technically accurate treatment) will improve the patient's physical status and be satisfying. Returning to health stability is satisfying and the purist physician does not have to consider organizational patient satisfaction motives to achieve this for a patient. Technically superior management based on expected outcomes should raise satisfaction. One simple example of this is the treatment of a UTI. Choosing the wrong antibiotic without understanding the local biogram of organism resistance will result in a higher likelihood of treatment failure, a patient's unhappy continuance of symptoms or worse, a worsening of status, which will lead to less satisfaction.

On communication, for the purposes of this discussion, the author defines communication as an unequal discussion between the physician and the patient with the emphasis on provision of explanations on the cause of illness, on the specific treatment components, on the treatment time period, and on the expectation of return to health. This is not purely unidirectional with the physician only speaking but a conversation between the two parties. Still the larger requirement of information provision and direction is on the physician. This can be contrasted with the initial interview as described above in which the physician benefits from *not speaking* unless providing open-ended encouraging questions ("Anything else?") such that the patient has uninterrupted opportunity to express concerns. The author acknowledges the issues of patient-centered treatment and mutual goal setting in respect of individualization, but is electing to focus on the technical aspect of communication including the explanation of the causes of a problem, test results and interpretation, projections of return to health and activity, and recourse if treatment failure.[32]

My fifth grade son is building a model of a lunar orbiter. I was reflecting and discussing with him about the real effort to build these devices, the technical effort to achieve a safe escape from the Earth's gravity and atmosphere and to protect from the freezing temperatures of space. I then mentioned it would be terrible to make technically weak landing equipment resulting in a crash and a project failure after all that effort and distance. About that time my son silently went out to ride his scooter.

Likewise, consider that physicians could work hard at listening to the patient's concerns, limit interruptions, determine a probable diagnosis, potentially confirm it with efficient use of testing, and align an appropriate intervention (with in the emergency department initiating some care), only to risk implementation failure once the patient was discharged. Consider your time and effort to assist this typical patient; this would leave *you* less than satisfied.

Regardless of whether this pleases a patient (though usually it does) and regardless of whether the patient returns to the hospital or clinic or emergency department as a return client (a business motive and thus repeated revenue benefit), the physician has a professional obligation (the correctness motive) to leverage a higher probability of attaining the expected health outcome once the patient is discharged. This is as important as knowing the correct evidence-based treatment as it is a technique of treatment. Unfortunately though much can be done and controlled within the emergency department, once treatment is to be continued at discharge, control can be and is often lost.

Adherence could be defined as the "extent to which a person's behavior – taking medication, following a diet, and/or executing lifestyle changes, corresponds with agreed recommendations from a health care provider."[44] To this end, the definition involves physician action(s); therefore, the performance of these participants must be considered within this text.

The implementation of and adherence to the treatment plan is a complex, multifactorial process and a difficult goal to attain for health care regardless of the setting. Often in chronic conditions such as diabetic and hypertensive management, the adherence average is only 50%.[44] In the acute setting adherence may be similarly challenging. In one emergency department study, prescription filling was absent in 12% of patients[45] and 26% in another.[46] In a different study, antibiotic adherence, defined as filling a prescription within 24 hours of discharge and finishing the prescription in the expected time period, was 49%.[47] Still another component, follow-up appointment attendance was 67%.[45] And overall, 33% of return visits were due to noncompliance with treatment plans.[48] All these rates are unfavorable to achieve consistent outcomes.

There are several factors or dimensions that impact treatment adherence, and these dimensions can be grouped as socioeconomic, health system, condition-related, therapy-related, and patient-related factors.[44] Since the ABEM's focus within the Communication/Professionalism requirement is on physician behavior, we will try to identify those technical factors related to physician activity that could be considered for potentiating more adherence. Based on the above described complexity and the resultant small aspect in overall adherence that emergency physicians appear to impact,[49] it is fortunate that the ABEM recognizes adherence as a multifactorial process and limits the individual APP C/P requirements to observation without an improvement requirement.

Uniquely within the health system, the environment of emergency medicine and patient interaction may predispose to poor methods of event closure and discharge. The activity of EM is usually single event care: Both parties recognize (hope) that the interaction will be once and not in a continuum especially if the patient has a primary care physician. Thus there is a tendency to relinquish or transpose responsibility for patient outcomes onto the future and ongoing interaction of the PCP.[50] Moreover, emergency medicine is associated with the time pressures of unscheduled patients who are potentially critically ill. It is a tendency of human nature toward time awareness to limit the time provided to current activities. Research on ED discharge communication often describes this incomplete interaction.[43] Striking is this resident study in which the length of time provided for discharge instructions was 76 seconds (range 7 to 202 seconds). Contrast this with a meta-analysis that shows increased adherence to a treatment plan when physicians are better communicators.[51] Understandably, the potential for operational change allowing emergency medicine physicians more time with patients is a balance of economic and technical outcome goals: the conflict of spending time with a current patient or moving on to a new patient.

Communication is not just about time length but also about content. Within the EM patient satisfaction literature, Sun et al identified four components of the exit discussion that patients were expecting and disappointed in not receiving including an explanation of the cause of illness or pain, an explanation of the test results, when to resume normal activity and when to return to the facility in the event of worsening.[32] In a study of hospital discharges, RNs provided more comprehensive discharge instruction than physicians.[52] In a study with emergency medicine residents, only 67% of the observed patients received complete discharge instructions/discussion including the above components,[43] and in a recent study a similar percentage of discharged emergency patients had poor comprehension of the instructions after discussion.[53] The lack of complete discharge instructions could result in less comprehension and thus less adherence.[54] Referring forward to the ABEM C/P requirement, one key assessment component is providing information including explaining the clinical impression and anticipated management course, providing information about tests and procedures, and giving the patient options.

Related to both the patient-related factors and health system factors, many EMRs or discharge programs provide information on the diagnosis and treatment at literacy levels beyond the patient's ability including a specific health or medical literacy.[55] Understandably, the choice and use of the EMR are more operational factors and outside of the individual physician's control; increased time may have to be applied to modifying the template discharge instructions at a compromise to the next patient and overall flow. Still, using simplified language (sixth grade level or less), nontechnical language, and using the patient's own language are associated with increased comprehension and are well within the realm of individual control.[55] This topic is a very challenging and complex issue and is beyond this discussion. The CMS Web site has provided a significant focus on the use of language in health care instructions and informational material.[56] Still another component of the ABEM C/P assessment is whether the physician used an appropriate language level.

The socioeconomic (SE) factors of adherence often compromise emergency medicine patient care as "low socioeconomic status may put patients in the position of having to choose between competing priorities."[44,57] Many EM patients have several of the SE factors that impact adherence including limited resources that must be shared with other family members and children, illiteracy, low level of education, unemployment, lack of effective social support networks and family dysfunction, unstable living conditions, and limits to access due to distance, cost of transport, or lack of transportation.[44,58,59] Most of these ills are beyond the emergency physician clinical reach during the singular visit and interaction, and it is valuable for the physician to recognize these factors and minimize exacerbating them with select treatment decisions.[60] Generalized examples of these potentially helpful actions are choosing a less expensive, equally effective medication and providing work excuses limiting the potential of job loss.

This section of Chapter 4 will be a brief introduction to one component of the American Board of Medical Specialties (ABMS) and the American Board of Emergency Medicine (ABEM) Maintenance of Certification (MOC) requirement, the Assessment of Practice Performance Communication/Professionalism (C/P) requirement, since it is aligned as above with the "hard quality" subject of the text. This section of Chapter 4 will describe the board certification requirement including the component of APP and provide specific discussion and an outline of the requirement for individual board-certified emergency physicians. The chapter will finish with suggestions of APP C/P foci that could be used by a physician to complete the APP requirement.

■ WHAT IS APP?

APP is one approach by the ABMS to encourage the application of the knowledge-based material (LLSA, etc) into clinical practice. The assessment of practice performance is the fourth component of the ABMS continuous learning process, with licensure, LLSA testing, and the certification (or recertification) examination as the other components (Table 4a-1).[2] The emphasis of the APP is on the application of the knowledge examined through the LLSA and examinations.

Part IV—Practice Performance Assessment

They are evaluated in their clinical practice according to specialty-specific standards for patient care. They are asked to demonstrate that they can assess the quality of care they provide compared to peers and national benchmarks and then apply the best evidence or consensus recommendations to improve that care using follow-up assessments.[2]

The two components of the ABEM's APP are the Patient Care Practice Improvement Activity (PCPI) and the Communication/Professionalism (C/P) patient feedback program. This section will focus on the Communication/Professionalism activity.

Reviewing the ABEM Web site on APP, the requirements for C/P activity will vary according to the board certification year and status of the physician. In general, the ABEM requires one C/P activity over the first 5 years and a second over the subsequent 5 years of the 10-year period between recertification (Figure 4b-4).

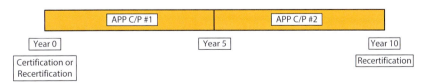

FIGURE 4B-4. General representation of APP C/P activity and board certification.

The APP PCPI requirement discussed in Chapter 4A has a similar time structure to its requirement. A physician, when in doubt about his or her requirements, can easily log in to the ABEM Web site, which has a well-formatted tracking system.

Unlike the APP PCPI requirement, the ABEM does not require a standard process improvement format (similar to PDSA) when completing the C/P activity. Instead the ABEM recommends assessing 10 patients on their experience and interaction with the physician without defining an improvement goal. Unlike the APP PCPI requirement the C/P process does not require a reassessment of 10 other patients to determine if practice change has occurred. The only requirement after completing the survey on 10 patients is to attest to the activity on the ABEM Web site. Moreover, the ABEM does not distinguish a preferred method or survey type:

> *Diplomates may use any formal method of assessing communication skills including patient surveys, interviews, or focus groups, administered at the institutional, departmental, or individual level. Some patient feedback methods that may meet ABEM requirements include Press-Ganey, CAHPS/ HCAHPS, and MAPPS. However, not all hospitals use a patient experience of care survey. ABEM has developed a survey form that is an adaptation of the CAHPS Clinician and Group Survey and Reporting Kit 2008.*[61]

Most hospitals are tracking patient satisfaction and are using one of the above survey tools. The physician should contact his or her medical director and inquire whether he or she can obtain some of the returned surveys. If the physician chooses to not use a hospital survey, the ABEM provides a patient experience of care survey form, which can be downloaded and used to fulfill their ABEM MOC APP Communication/Professionalism requirement. From a procedural approach, if the individual physician is managing the survey, he or she should consider the methods of surveys. Among other issues, the physician will need to consider whether the survey should be completed during the ED visit (presumably after discharge) or as a separate event once the patient has left the facility. The logistics are different in each case and the physician may have to include a larger sample of patients to receive 10 completed surveys in the latter situation (many outpatient surveys achieve low completion rates).

The ABEM defines the assessment requirements with a categorization of the physician behavior.[61] A minimum of one physician behavior must be measured from each of the following three categories:

1. Communications/listening, for example
   - Communicate clearly with patients and other medical staff by listening carefully and couching language at the appropriate level for the listener.
2. Providing information, for example
   - Explain the clinical impression and anticipated management course to the patient and the patient's family.

- Provide information about tests and procedures.
- Give the patient options.

3. Showing concern for the patient, for example
   - Show respect to the patient and other medical staff.
   - Make the patient feel comfortable by asking if they have any questions or concerns and act to address their concerns.
   - Ask the patient about adequate pain relief.

Many of the suggested tools would have questions that meet the above three categories and thus can be used for efficient completion of the requirement.

Considering the prolonged introduction of this chapter relation to the three categories, the technically focused emergency physician can incorporate the technically-oriented goals and still be compliant with the patient satisfaction requirement. With Category #1 above, *listening carefully* can be extended to listening for a longer time without interrupting the patient. Category #1 could lead to a heightened level of clinical diagnosis while being a satisfier. It also involves the appropriate level of language. With Category #2, the discussion on communication reinforces the goals of successful implementation of a treatment course and adherence to the treatment plans (including three of four components of discharge instructions). With Category #3, focusing on symptom relief not just pain relief is a standard goal with patient management as well as utilizing the concept of open questions ("Anything else?") during the interview and visit conclusion that could encourage the patient to share his or her medical concerns.

■ ATTESTATION

After completing the survey, diplomates should attest that they have completed a patient feedback activity to meet the Communication/Professionalism requirement. The ABEM APP C/P requirement is not requiring evidence of a practice change. Attestation is to affirm the physician has 10 patient surveys involved in the three categories.

On the ABEM website is the Patient Experience of Care Survey that the ABEM developed from the AHRQ CAHPS tool. This is a good tool in regards to the clinical or technical focus advocated in this text. Several questions focus on listening, open questioning, communications about the diagnosis, and treatment plan.

In conclusion, it is important to carefully review and understand the goals of patient satisfaction; the business motives must be held separate of the clinical goals.[38] The priority focus must be on our technical quality with the consideration of service elements that may align with technical processes that could leverage clinical outcomes. The individual provider and the medical staff must be steadfast advocates for the Institute of Medicine's aims focusing on technical accuracy and efficiency that balance an administration's approach to hospitality. It is notable that the Institution of Medicine's six aims do not include patient satisfaction, only centeredness—a very different item.[62] We have not achieved the Institute of Medicine's six aims to any significant level. Perhaps we should focus on these, achieving a higher technical outcomes and error-free care.

REFERENCES

1. Nelson RN. Demystifying maintenance of certification. *Ann Emerg Med.* 2014;467-470.

2. American Board of Medical Specialties. *MOC Competencies and Criteria.* Chicago, IL: ABMS; August 4, 2014.

3. American Board of Emergency Medicine. *MOC Assessment of Practice Performance (APP) Overview.* East Lansing, MI: ABEM; August 4, 2014.

4. American Board of Emergency Medicine. *Maintenance of Certification (MOC) Policies and Procedures.* East Lansing, MI: ABEM; 2014.

5. American Board of Emergency Medicine. *A Primer on ABEM MOC APP Practice Improvement Requirements.* East Lansing, MI: ABEM; August 4, 2014.

6. Brennan TA. The role of physician specialty board certification status in the quality movement. *JAMA.* 2004;1038-1043.

7. Jamtvedt G, Young JM, Kristoffersen DT, O'Brien MA, Oxman AD. Does telling people what they have been doing change what they do? A systematic review of the effects of audit and feedback. *Qual Saf Health Care.* 2006;433-436.

8. American College of Emergency Physicians. Continuing education: assessment of practice performance. *ACEP.* 2014, August 6. www.acep.org.

9. American Board of Medical Specialties. *Standards for the ABMS Program for Maintenance of Certification (MOC).* Chicago, IL: ABMS; 2014.

10. Huff JS, Melnick ER, Tomaszewski CA, et al. Clinical policy: critical issues in the evaluation and management of adult patients presenting to the emergency department with seizures. *Ann Emerg Med.* 2014;437-447.

11. ACEP. Practice parameter: neuroimaging in the emergency patient presenting with seizure. *Ann Emerg Med.* 1996;114-118.

12. Wolf SJ, Lo B, Shih RD, Smith MD, Fesmire FM; American College of Emergency Physicians Clinical Policies Committee. Clinical policy: critical issues in the evaluation and management of adult patients in the emergency department with asymptomatic elevated blood pressure. *Ann Emerg Med.* 2013;59-68.

13. Hahn SA, Lavonas EJ, Mace SE, Napoli AM, Fesmire FM; American College of Emergency Physicians Clinical Policies Subcommittee on Early Pregnancy. Clinical policy: critical issues in the initial evaluation and management of patients presenting to the emergency department in early pregnancy. *Ann Emerg Med.* 2012;60:381-390.

14. Barnhart KT. Ectopic pregnancy. *N Engl J Med.* 2009;361:379-387.

15. Fesmire FM, Brown MD, Espinosa JA, et al. Critical issues in the evaluation and management of adult patients presenting to the emergency department with suspected pulmonary embolism. *Ann Emerg Med.* 2011;628-652.

16. Howell JM, Eddy OL, Lukens TW, et al. Clinical policy: critical issues in the evaluation and management of emergency department patients with suspected appendicitis. *Ann Emerg Med.* 2010;55:71-116.

17. Hlibczuk V. Diagnostic accuracy of noncontrast computed tomography for appendicitis in adults: a systematic review. *AEM*. January 2010;51-59.

18. Thomas, S. Effects of morphine analgesia on diagnostic accuracy in emergency department patients with abdominal pain: a prospective, randomized trial. *J Am Coll Surg*. 2003;18-31.

19. Samaras, N. Older patients in the emergency department: a review. *Ann Emerg Med*. 2010;261-269.

20. Eldow JA, Panagos PD, Godwin SA, et al. Clinical policy: critical issues in the evaluation and management of adult patients presenting to the emergency department with acute headache. *Ann Emerg Med*. 2008;407-436.

21. Suarez JI, Tarr RW, Selman WR. Aneurysmal subarachnoid hemorrhage. *NEJM*. 2006;387-96.

22. McCormack RF, Hutson A. Can computed tomography angiography of the brain replace lumbar puncture in the evaluation of acute-onset headache after a negative noncontrast cranial computed tomography scan? *Acad Emerg Med*. 2010;444-451.

23. Connolly ES, Rabinstein AA, Carhuapoma JR , et al. Guidelines for the management of aneurysmal subarachnoid hemorrhage: a guideline for healthcare professionals from the American Heart Association/American Stroke Association. *Stroke*. 2012;1-39.

24. Huff JS, Decker WW, Quinn JV. Clinical policy: critical issues in the evaluation and management of adult patients presenting to the emergency department with syncope. *Ann Emerg Med*. 2007;431-444.

25. Quinn J, McDermott D. Electrocardiogram findings in emergency department patients with syncope. *Acad Emerg Med*. 2011;714-18.

26. Singh A, Alter HJ, Littlepage A. A systematic review of medical therapy to facilitate passage of ureteral calculi. *Ann Emerg Med*. 2007;552-563.

27. Abrahamian FM, K. A. Association of pyuria and clinical characteristics with the presence of urinary tract infection among patients with acute nephrolithiasis. *Ann Emerg Med*. 2013;526-533.

28. Teichman, J. M. Acute renal colic from ureteral calculus. *N Engl J Med*. 2004;684-93

29. American College of Radiology. Acute onset flank pain—suspicion of stone disease. Retrieved from http://www.acr.org/Quality-Safety/Appropriateness-Criteria 2011.

30. Abrahamian FM, Krishnadasan A, Mower WR, Moran GJ, Talan DA. Association of pyuria and clinical characteristics with the presence of urinary tract infection among patients with acute nephrolithiasis. *Ann Emerg Med*. 2013;62(5):526-533.

31. Farley H, Enguidanos ER, Coletti CM. Patient satisfaction surveys and quality of care: an information paper. *Ann Emerg Med*. 2014;351-357.

32. Sun BC. Determinants of patient satisfaction and willingness to return with emergency care. *Ann Emerg Med*. 2000;426-434.

33. Stearns CR. Antibiotic prescriptions are associated with increased patient satisfaction with emergency department visits for acute respiratory tract infections. *Acad Emerg Med*. 2009;934-941.

34. Fenton JJ, Jerant AF, Bertakis KD, Franks P. The cost of satisfaction. *Arch Intern Medicine*. 2012;405-411.

35. Kaplan J. Better clinical outcomes, patient satisfaction go hand in hand for emergency physicians. *ACEP Now*. April 11, 2014.

36. Arrow KJ. Uncertainty and the welfare economics of medical care. *Am Econ Rev*. 1963;941-973.

37. Bowers MR, Kiefe CI. Measuring health care quality: comparing and contrasting the medical and marketing approaches. *Am J Med Qual*. 2002;136-144.

38. Sequist TD, Schneider EC, Anastario M. Quality monitoring of physicians: linking patients' experiences of care to clinical quality and outcomes. *J Gen Intern Med*. 2008;1784-1790.

39. Peterson MC, Holbrook JH, Hales D. Contributions of the history, physical examination, and laboratory investigation in making medical diagnoses. *West J Medicine*. 1992;163-165.

40. Hampton JR. Relative contributions of history-taking, physical examination, and laboratory investigation to diagnosis and management of medical outpatients. *Br Med J*. 1975;486-489.

41. Marvel MK, Epstein RM, Flowers K, Beckman HB. Soliciting the patient's agenda: have we improved? *JAMA*. 1999;283-287.

42. Rabinowitz I. Length of patient's monologue, rate of completion, and relation to other components of the clinical encounter. *Br Med J*. 2004;501-502.

43. Rhodes KV. Resuscitating the physician-patient relationship: emergency department communication in an academic medical center. *Ann Emerg Med*. 2004;262-267.

44. World Health Organization. *Adherence to Long-Term Therapies*. Geneva: WHO; 2003.

45. Thomas EJ. Patient noncompliance with medical advice after the emergency department visit. *Ann Emerg Med*. 1996;49-55.

46. Ding R, Zeger SL. The validity of self-reported primary adherence among medicaid patients discharged from the emergency department with a prescription medication. *Ann Emerg Med*. 2013;225-234.

47. Suffoletto B, Calabria J. A mobile phone text message program to measure oral antibiotic use and provide feedback on adherence to patients discharged from the emergency department. *Acad Emerg Med*. 2012;949-958.

48. Keith KD. Emergency department revisits. *Ann Emerg Med*. 1989;964-68.

49. Samuels-Kalow ME, Stack AM. Effective discharge communication in the emergency department. *Ann Emerg Med*. 2012;152-159.

50. Horwitz DA, Schwarz ES. Emergency department patients with diabetes have better glycemic control when they have identifiable primary care providers. *Acad Emerg Med*. 2012;650-655.

51. Haskard Zolnierek KB, DiMatteo MR. Physician communication and patient adherence to treatment: a meta-analysis. *Med Care*. 2009;826-834.

52. Ashbrook L, Mourad M. Communicating discharge instructions to patients: a survey of nurse, intern, and hospitalist practices. *J Hosp Med*. 2003;36-41.

53. Musso MW. Patients' comprehension of their emergency department encounter: a pilot study using physician observers. *Ann Emerg Med*. 2014;1-5.

54. Engel KG, Heisler M. Patient comprehension of emergency department care and instructions: are patients aware of when they do not understand? *Ann Emerg Med.* 2009;454-461.

55. Spandorfer JM. Comprehension of discharge instructions by patients in an urban emergency department. *Ann Emerg Med.* 1995;71-74.

56. CMS. Toolkit for making written material clear and effective. September 29, 2014. http://www.cms.gov/Outreach-and-Education/Outreach/WrittenMaterialsToolkit/index.html.

57. Stevens TB, Richmond NL. Prevalence of nonmedical problems among older adults presenting to the emergency department. *Acad Emerg Med.* 2014;651-658.

58. Suffoletto B, Yealy DM. The trouble with medication adherence after emergency care. *Ann Emerg Med.* 2013;235-236.

59. McCarthy ML, Ding R. Does providing prescription information or services improve medication adherence among patients discharged from the emergency department? a randomized controlled trial. *Ann Emerg Med.* 2013;212-223.

60. Blanchard J, Madden JM. The relationship between emergency department use and cost-related medication nonadherence among medicare beneficiaries. *Ann Emerg Med.* 2013;475-485.

61. ABEM. Communication/professionalism activity. *ABEM.* September 11, 2014. www.abem.org.

62. Institute of Medicine. *Crossing the Quality Chasm.* Washington, DC: National Academy Press; 2001.

Implementing a Sequential Clinical Auditing Program

In prior chapters, I described the challenges of the current physician review systems. In Chapter 3, I introduced the sequential clinical auditing program that I think addresses the gaps of the current programs. The idea may have intrigued you; unfortunately merely describing these issues will not implement a program within your practice realm.

Sequential clinical auditing is about changing culture through changing processes and knowledge. The current way physicians monitor physician practice performance is poor. There needs to be a different way. Sequential clinical auditing (SCA) is a method that addresses the weaknesses of current programs while aligning groups with future value-focused health care change. The menu or script for SCA in this book is straightforward, but it is only part of the solution. The other "stuff" is the work of leading change in physician organizations. I will use *Leading Change*[1] and the Eight Common Errors as a platform of discussion. Another good source is the AHRQ's Technical Review titled, "Closing the Quality Gap: A Critical Analysis of Quality Improvement Strategies Volume 1—Series Overview and Methodology," which provides a review of the QI theories that are currently employed in health care change. SCA is a strategy for cultural change (described within this chapter) which can be viewed within the larger theory of health care QI.[2]

A first step will be to assess your group's readiness. This also pertains to moving from one audit, in sequence to another audit topic, or not. It is my experience that most groups could be defined into four categories: in a temporary steady state; in decline or stagnation in which the individual needs predominate group structure; in a reactionary state, fight or flight behaviors from contract disputes, poor quality and risk management issues; and aggressively improving, or expanding (looking outward at the market) and introspective (looking inward at the quality of group practice). Figure 5-1 represents this spectrum of group status.

Most groups struggle between stability and reactionary behavior. There are bright spots dependent on some physicians and leaders, though others are not engaged in the group process. Individual work maintains the level of quality and

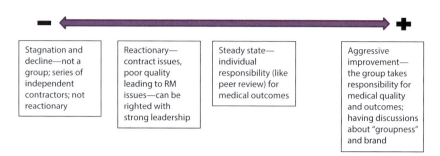

FIGURE 5-1. The spectrum of group status.

outcomes, which is probably due to hiring well and attracting good talent. Much like many organizations, there is complacency. Past successes of achieving medical school, achieving residency with or without fellowship, achieving that top income, and being involved in daily, one-on-one care have often resulted in an inability to visualize crises. The demands of CMS and TJC are leveled at the institution such that each facility then must make requests of physician practice change; the physician response is to claim a loss of autonomy and hopeful ignoring of some reasonable albeit anemic requirements. The low performance standards that a medical staff promote in hospitals are an example of the complacency, and the result is a rare management of poor technical practice. In the end, the physician can argue away his technical inadequacies, report he or she is doing "what is required," and remain status quo. He or she cannot see his or her practice atrophying.

If there is no crisis, there is minimal need for change. If the administration is not happy with the group and is requesting a contract review or a competitor just built a stand-alone ED within the new development in the same town as your facility or if the current peer review system (unlikely) somehow triggered on a series of medical events that question the technical ability of several of the group's physicians then it is hard to combat the inertia with a large process change. Physicians are as good at denial as most people; I was with a group that had a contract challenge and they were appalled that others were questioning their clinical quality. Of course they had nothing to show that they were better or even to show that they were managing quality (at the time). Unfortunately, if these issues have not occurred within your group … they will.

A group in the reactionary status is not at the level or stability to initiate SCA. The physicians will be concerned about the newness and will only interpret the method as another act that threatens their livelihood and professional status. You should be looking to assist with stabilization first and weathering the crisis and then over time to encourage consideration of SCA.

If you then consider "creating the crisis" this will probably result in your head. I am not aware of any chair or medical director who is willing to create stress within the physician group in order to create change. Bombarding physicians with unachievable operational metrics is inadequate; most physicians look upon the metrics as external manipulations for cost control (or revenue enhancement by

CMGs) rather than for medical quality and market share. Talking about a competitor's movements and the market is numbing for physicians who have minimal experience in this and minimal interest (some emergency physicians especially would consider another party taking away some of the exhausting patients and their demands as positive!). In the end, though the leader recognizes the crisis perhaps overt action will not be successful. A less dramatic gradual method described later in this chapter could have success.

When introducing SCA into groups with stability, you need to assess the status of key individual members. Junior members may be going through board preparation and have many external demands, whereas senior members may have less interest since they may be considering a closure to their career. As with any change, creating a guiding coalition is important. Unfortunately, within emergency physician groups with average size of 12-15 members, this limits the size of the "coalition" to perhaps yourself and another two members (Figure 5-2). Still, if you are not in a leadership position then the first member to recruit should be the medical director or chair. Power roles are necessary in early development though influence takes over in time. Identify "early adopters" but avoid the new physicians (just out of residency) in the group as they have no clout yet and potentially you can damage their career and the implementation allowing their zeal to represent the process. Instead, look for three physician leaders (often well-spoken and "senior" doctors with a vision outside of the institution) and speak with them about the value of the program. They will be the anchors of the group's culture and you will have to address the potential disruption; there will be questions of partnership and livelihood threat, administration exposure, cost, and in general an explanation of why (give them this book). Be willing to accept a trial period for the program which may be their wishful response that the new idea will die over time (depends on your dedication and energy).

A "sensible" vision will "direct, align, and inspire actions" with the group.[1] My simple statement on one initiative was "the group must support the individual such that the individual can support the group through clinical practice"

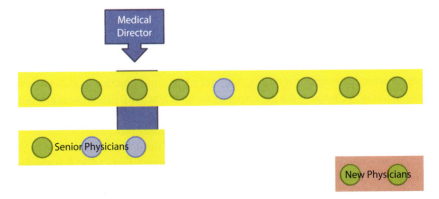

FIGURE 5-2. Coalition members within the group (blue dots).

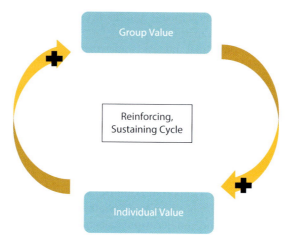

FIGURE 5-3. A simple vision.

(Figure 5-3). This is nonconfrontational and works. The statement promotes a mutually supportive relationship.

Interesting is to view this vision with today's groups. CMGs and independent contracts often minimally "invest" in the individual though these businesses promote compliance and risk programs, scheduling programs, and Web-based libraries as support. Real investing is a group's committed internal program to continual member assessment and raising a member's technical accuracy or quality that affirms the member's commitment to the group.

Repeating the above simple statement, "the group must support the individual such that the individual can support the group through clinical practice," promotes acceptance. The repetition reinforces the vision that this was a positive change and will help physicians with their primary task: providing better medical care. As usual, words followed by actions are more successful than words alone. Implementing the sequential clinical audits and producing the first summary is essential to reinforce that vision. The value of SCA is the sequence, not just for improvement in clinical practice which is the primary goal, but also for cultural change. Employee behavior patterns with process change resist the new change or initially conform but then revert to old methods. With the repetitive pattern of SCA, the process is continual which physicians cannot ignore. Continual review and practice modification is not mammoth change, but a quiet month-to-month activity. The communication of the audits, the summaries, and the discussion within the group via e-mail or meetings maintains the vision and promotes the ongoing process.

In many ways, introducing the SCA method into the group is similar to *Kairyo* in Japanese quality management, whereas the ongoing activity of SCA is similar to *Kaizen*.[3] Though Kairyo is a large step and initiated usually through a few committed champions, the Kaizen of SCA is the monthly, total-group engagement and small-step continual change (Figure 5-4). As mentioned previously, once the

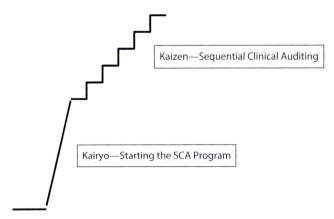

FIGURE 5-4. Kairyo to Kaizen process.

group becomes fully engaged, the technique becomes culture and the group drives the repetitive process. As for the leader (yourself), you become more transparent, becoming the medium and the process influences individual change. As the group process (culture) becomes stronger, you may reduce your power presence.

Once the inertia has broken, the pace of the activity must be monitored. Two rate limiters are involved with SCA. First, the method and rate of abstraction is important to producing the frequent early audit wins that will impact the physicians in the group. Reliance on personnel to mine the data makes you dependent on other's productivity and work quality. Fortunately you can create your deadlines and amend them but the sequential production must be ensured. The repetitive nature of the auditing modifies the culture. Second, monitoring the physician acceptance and incorporation of the audit findings is necessary. Expect some resistance as the physicians in the group should objectively and subjectively provide both individual and group review of the data. Judging the resistance to the data and the recommendations may encourage you to slow the delivery of the subsequent audit, thus allowing for more review, perhaps another presentation or more one-on-one conversations, and consideration. Some groups will be slower in acceptance based on the composition of the members. The cyclic aspect of auditing will allow a future review and another opportunity to modify practice. Practice change is the goal, not your own productivity.

It may take a while for all physicians to accept the program. A colleague stopped me in the hospital hallway one day and said, "Tony, I think I can finally support you in this program and the money we are paying you." That statement was 2 years and many audits after I had initiated the program! I thanked her. I had not questioned her commitment. It shows that some individuals can silently resist for long periods and each individual has a threshold.

If you are a junior leader in your organization, you will need to communicate more frequently with the chair or medical director on the steps and activities of the SCA program. First, the director or chair can amplify your voice and increase the frequency of the message; moreover, the leader is usually one of the senior physicians in the group and overt acceptance of the SCA program will encourage others to accept. Third, the leader has the opportunity to promote the activity within the institution and achieve a secondary goal. Promoting the group's clinical quality is valuable for contract stability and essential for medical staff relations; the leader has interactions with the CMO, CEO, and the medical staff president. Providing the leader with first access to the data, even prepping with an "elevator speech" is not wrong just practical.

There are relatively few overt obstacles when implementing SCA. Structurally, you must ensure that the information, in multimedia form, is distributed to the recipients, the physicians. Most groups have monthly departmental meetings; often reviewing the most recent audit results and having a discussion become secondary to other "hot" departmental crises, such as administrative complaints, financial information, etc. At times you must battle to keep this on the agenda. Though other methods of communication are essential, maintaining the feedback loop of the audit process and embedding it within current culture is critical (ironically, as described in the text—auditing for improving clinical accuracy should improve financial status and reduce administrative complaints!). Strong groups realize the primacy of clinical work and learn to value the feedback but can be distracted with other less direct concerns.

Addressing the mechanics of performing SCA becomes an issue of skills and time. Physicians should stay practicing medicine and the group should hire data abstractors. Employing (premedical) students from the local college enables you remain a director, focusing on the structure and the message and not only on data management and analysis.

You should choose simple attainable audits first. You should choose large volume or high frequency, noncontroversial topics to produce audits for the first year. Your major obstacle as mentioned above is communication. Maintain a monthly meeting presence, but also commit to one-on-one conversations. Fortunately the physician groups are small enough to allow for this. For one group, I had a goal of a conversation a week which allowed four conversations per physician-colleague annually, not including the individual audit feedback or departmental meeting discussions. This pattern seemed to keep everyone aware of the activity. Moreover, during those conversations I would be asking for feedback, encouraging the physicians to direct the process with ideas and clinical topics. The goal was engagement and ownership and contrasted with the external reviews that are deemed punitive and threats to the physician status.

The hospital administration may inquire about the SCA activity. This is understandable, the medical director or chair should be selectively "mentioning" the clinical strength of the group during C-suite activities. Still this is a precarious position, and a CMO request to meet and discuss the data or to present at the hospital quality committee or in a grand round presentation has the potential to undermine the efforts of introduction and cultural change within the physician group. First, if you are not the medical director or chair, your presentation could be looked upon as a power move and you would lose the interest of your most valuable champion(s).

Second, the physician group might have angst about public data exposure without being present during the presentation. If you are given no choice, one way to address this is to accept the public presentation, such as a grand round presentation, but introduce the method only and limit or "whitewash" the results. Moreover, present the data with the physician group in attendance so there can be no question of intent. In the past, I avoided these presentations and let the medical director or chair work different levels and channels. It is most important to develop the "roots" of SCA in the physician culture—attend to your colleagues and not your career.

Celebrate and market the wins. The repetitive pattern of SCA predisposes to wins. A win is a strong culture establisher. There is nothing stronger to enhance acceptance that the SCA process will help practice than a physician observing that he or she is practicing well. The beauty about much of this data is that the negatives are often positives depending on the perspective (clinical appreciative inquiry!). Consider an audit on abdominal pain and the use of serum lipase to assess for pancreatitis. If the data showed that the physicians obtained a serum lipase with a frequency at 85% but all pancreatitis patients were identified, then celebrate the consistency and completeness of the evaluation. Unfortunately this might be overuse, misuse, or underuse, but a single data point in the process can be viewed from many directions (Figure 5-5). How you manage the next steps is a strength of the process. Through a group discussion and review of the literature, the group could decide to reduce the frequency of serum lipase testing while maintaining a goal of 100% first-presentation identification of pancreatitis. The group enacts a process change within the department. The subsequent audit shows a reduction in serum lipase frequency to 25% but all pancreatitis cases were identified. Celebrate this win as well. This is the value of sequential clinical auditing—repetition allows

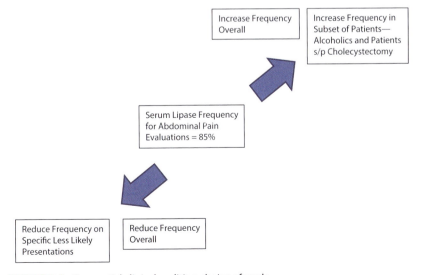

FIGURE 5-5. Sequential clinical auditing choice of goals.

for the identification of improvement and short-term wins. Gains in the primary physician activity allow for the cultural process establishment. [Note: The irony about medical practice is that much of our activity has no comparative data and few benchmarks such that you can establish group or local standards through the use of EBM and then start a process improvement (see standard of care comment in Chapter 2)]. Talking up the wins at many levels is important; give the medical director or chair the opportunity to share and give the physicians in the group their successes.

Usually physicians do not view the group structure and management activity as a method of improvement. The sensible vision as mentioned above allows the physicians within the group to realize that a department or group can be more than a "holding company" dealing only in reimbursement or compliance but an actual organization that could enable better outcomes through its processes. Frequently showing the practice change is a simple reinforcement of the tool, SCA, and modifies the participants' acceptance. This cannot be passive. The SCA activity must have presence on every departmental agenda, every audit and its results must be internally promoted, and the director or mediator for the SCA process must be dedicated to physician interaction and communication in order to actively anchor the process within culture. There is no finish line, but when the physicians in the group start directing and/or giving suggestions for audits, that is a positive milestone; individually he or she has incorporated the program into his or her realm of practice and is becoming engaged and reliant on it. Expectation is but one victory.

There is a lot of talk about disruption in organizations. SCA is not a disruptive process when made compatible with the genes of the physician group. In this text, there have been descriptions of various EM physician groups and from the start you must recognize the status of the group. From my experience, those groups with the most "group" or collective presence or culture and who often have an innate understanding that the group's brand represents high quality to the community are more apt to recognize and incorporate SCA methods (these are often the aggressive, improving groups). Independent contractor groups are often weak in culture and thus less able to institute a program, though it should and can be achieved locally.

REFERENCES

1. Kotter JP. *Leading Change*. Boston, MA: Harvard Business School Press; 1996.

2. Agency for Healthcare Research and Quality. *Closing the Quality Gap: A Critical Analysis of Quality Improvement Strategies Volume 1—Series Overview and Methodology*. Rockville, MD: AHRQ; 2004.

3. Galgano A. *Companywide Quality Management*. Portland, OR: Productivity Press; 1994.

Closure and Continuance

Recently I overheard an EM physician, "a colleague" due to our mutual specialty, try to explain to the hospitalist service his reason for admitting a patient. He was getting pushback from the hospitalist because he has a pattern in which the logic and science behind his arguments are poor. It was not the first time this has happened and I have heard the hospitalists complain (individuals I highly regard).

This physician appears to be the nicest person: He has a great game face for customer service (I know him only professionally), he spends large quantities of time at the bedside, and I suspect he scores well in patient satisfaction. He even cares about other physicians, handing out philosophical sayings to several of us. Apparently I am in need of help … which I realize.

I suspect this physician is out of balance with his practice. Maybe he was never technically strong or more likely the system did not support his continued technical development after residency. The latter is more probable but often either are occurring or have occurred. The maintenance of technical competence is very challenging. Some of the important components are adequate volumes and acuity of patients, a breadth of pathology entering the ED, a personal commitment to introspection and continuous reflection, a program within the group that organizes review of practice and does not assume competency, all the way to some legislated competency like a license.

Maybe this physician always had the extra-professionalism approach. It is not wrong. But technical competence has to be present as well, and primarily. Patients want us to be correct not just friendly. Unfortunately some physicians recognize that charm (serving coffee) is a goal of the system (standard business marketing—it brings customers back).[1] Equally unfortunate, the current health care systems are often blind to varying technical ability and as described often assume the medical staff will manage the technical competence. Programs like peer review and core measure management are inadequate. The system is imbalanced as well and is not helping the individual.

This work is about resuming our responsibility for technical quality in health care such that we can right the imbalance currently allowing patient satisfaction elements to dominate the discussion of patient value and the grading of physicians. We need to move from perceived to hard components of quality, recognizing that

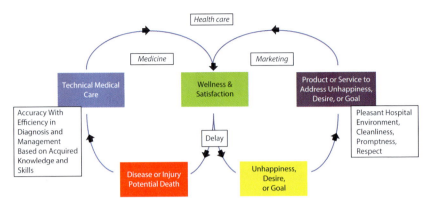

FIGURE 6-1. Simplified relationship between medical care and marketing (from Chapter 1).

marketing has its place in health care and technical accuracy and precision has its place in medical care (Figure 6-1).

In rebalancing, as we take increased responsibility for technical quality we need to realize the inadequacies of our systems of review and assessment. The JC FPPE and OPPE programs at each institution allow for standardization and compliance, a base form of quality, though such framework is not restrictive. Medical staffs could develop more comprehensive systems of practice review while achieving compliance. Each department or institution could work with its PR components be it the entry triggers, the timing of throughput and feedback, and the combination of patient complaints and system issues. The incorporation of EB literature in addition to experience-based review/critique allows for a stronger alignment with expected outcomes and supports a physician's movement toward practice change (Figure 6-2). Peer review overall has to be the balance of physician support and patient support and a transparent group process. Still, peer review does not provide an adequate sample size for representation of the volume and breadth of an EM physician's practice. It also has a limited feedback to other group members as a learning method (Table 6-1). Despite this, the untapped worth of a peer review

■ TABLE 6-1. Comparison of Hard Quality Review Processes

Variable	Standard Peer Review	Sequential Clinical Audit	Assessment of Practice Performance PCPI
Sample size/representation	Small	Mid to large	Small
Represents breadth of specialty	No	Yes	No
Individual focus	Yes	Yes	Yes
Group focus	No	Yes	No
Can differentiate a group or physician	No	Yes	No

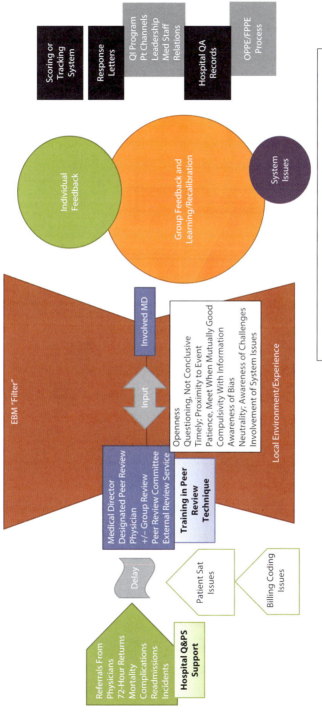

FIGURE 6-2. Summary of the peer review process.

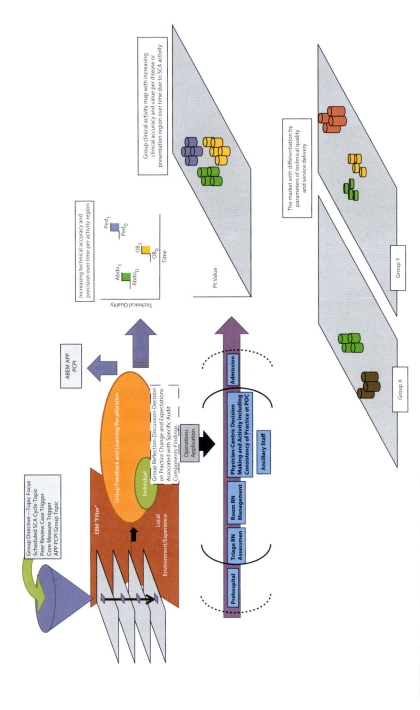

FIGURE 6-3. Overall physician performance linkage.

program becomes more evident when combined with a program such as SCA, moving from quality assurance and reactivity to a larger more comprehensive review and proactive opportunity for improvement.

Similar to PR the ABEM APP PCPI requirement is a minor demand on board-certified physicians. Alas, we must jump through hoops though the components of the process such as cyclic review for practice change and the allowance of focus choice on a disease process or a chief complaint can be positive. Having the APP PCPI incorporated and produced through a SCA program would potentially achieve more value for physicians (Table 6-1).

Sequential clinical auditing is a more comprehensive, transparent, translational, impactful program (Figure 6-3). The value of SCA comes from its sampling and feedback pattern which being sequential, ongoing and cyclic is distinct from the randomness of PR and the infrequency of APP PCPI processes (Table 6-1). Moreover, SCA can be incorporative of PR, APP, and core measure work. The findings from an audit affect individual and group clinical activity, allow the group to direct local practice activity within their "shop," and can impact operations through less waste, less rework, and higher capacity. An SCA program has the potential to differentiate the group within the market that PR and CM compliance cannot achieve. SCA can represent an institution's brand.

We are finished; I hope I have provided an appealing argument for how I see the world. Writing is a daunting process; one can only try to capture a time point in the status of a system and that the description harmonizes with other material, justifies the effort of the reader and reflector, and extends the conversation further. Hopefully this material will add to the knowledge and commitment of others and can assist organizations in the dialogue and incorporation of methods to achieve a higher technical quality of practice. The SCA program is one method of focusing on an individual physician's and a group's technical quality allowing for a rebalancing of focus in health care that more consistently addresses a patient's needs.

REFERENCE

1. Welch S. Service recovery boosts customer loyalty and patient satisfaction. *Emergency Medicine News*. August 2012;34(8):9.

Index